BENT

BUT NOT

BROKEN

ONE FAMILY'S SCOLIOSIS JOURNEY

BENT
BUT NOT
BROKEN

ONE FAMILY'S SCOLIOSIS JOURNEY

ANDREW
BUTTERS

WITH AVERY BUTTERS
& JODI WILKS-BUTTERS

MEATH

OGHMA CREATIVE MEDIA

www.oghmacreative.com

ISBN: 978-1-63373-338-1

Interior Design by Casey W. Cowan
Editing by Gordon Bonnet

Meath Press
Oghma Creative Media
Bentonville, Arkansas
www.oghmacreative.com

For scoliosis kids and families everywhere.

CONTENTS

PROLOGUE

MY LITTLE STANLEY CUP

June 13, 2002. Three weeks before my wife Jodi's due date of July 4th. I was always a bit ticked at that because, being Canadian, July 1st is our national birthday and it would have been cool for our daughter to share that date with Confederation.

Being Canadian also meant that I was following the National Hockey League playoffs. Jodi and I had just watched the final game across the street with our friends, Trevor and Iza. The Detroit Red Wings won and in the grand tradition of the sport, after the Stanley Cup was presented to the team captain, Steve Yzerman, he hoisted it above his head and then lowered it to his face so he could plant a big kiss on it. My father received two offers to join the Red Wings back in the 50s. He declined both, but that organization has always held a special place with me.

As we lay in bed that night, Jodi and I engaged in the usual bedtime kisses and instead of reaching for her hand to hold as I fell asleep I rolled onto my side and patted Jodi on the belly. "Okay, you can give birth now," I said. We both laughed and went to sleep.

Early the next morning, earlier than I needed to be awake for work, Jodi woke me by standing at the side of the bed and nudging my shoulder. "Andrew," she said, "we're going to have a baby."

"I know," I replied and rolled back over.

"No. we're going to have a baby TODAY. My water just broke."

I jumped out of bed like someone had pulled the fire alarm and started scrambling to get ready. We didn't have a go-bag put together or anything, and we needed to put some clothes into a duffle and then make the thirty-minute drive down the highway to the hospital where Jodi was born and where her mom worked as a nurse.

Jodi let me scramble around for a bit before informing me that she wasn't in labor and we had some time to have a shower and get ready before we had to leave. The pregnancy classes failed to inform me that:

a) The water can break without the woman being in labor; and

b) Once the water breaks you have about 24 hours to give birth or…
I don't know. Something else happens.

It's possible that instead of not being informed, maybe I wasn't paying attention in the classes.

So after we got ready, we packed up the car and went to head out. Trevor and Iza were also about to have a baby. In fact, Iza's due date was right around that day. We ran into Trevor, who was walking the dog and he asked us if we were going to the cottage for the weekend. Jodi explained that we were going to have a baby. Well, I guess Iza heard what was going on and poked her head out of her upstairs window to get some clarification.

Jodi confirmed the news, but I won't repeat what Iza said here. Suffice it to say she wasn't thrilled with the idea of still being pregnant while Jodi got to go give birth.

We drove to Woodstock, Ontario to Jodi's childhood home, and dropped in to see her dad and give him his Father's Day present a couple days early. He had the same look on his face that I had when Jodi told him not to worry, that we had time to spare.

We were pre-registered at the hospital so we went straight to the maternity ward where a doctor that was not Jodi's came to talk to us to get us squared away. We hadn't called ahead or anything so the fact that Jodi's doctor wasn't at the hospital wasn't a surprise.

Then, Jodi's mom showed up and told us Jodi's doctor was in the hospital. This is great, we thought, she won't have to make a special trip in to deliver the baby. Well, it turned out that Jodi's doctor was a *patient* in the hospital. She had suffered a heart attack and was currently downstairs recovering.

That was curveball Number One.

Curveball Number Two came when the doctor informed us that he was on vacation as of seven o'clock that night. Oh, and Jodi's parents were supposed to go see Cyndi Lauper and Cher in Toronto, a ninety-minute drive down the highway, that night.

We had to decide on what to do.

Options included:

a) Waiting it out to see what happened. If labour hadn't started by sometime that afternoon we'd have to travel to London and have the baby there;

b) Decide right now to go to London and let everything play out as it plays out; or

c) Start an IV drip of the magic labor-inducing liquid and get 'er dun as quickly as possible, hopefully before the good doctor had to make tracks and get out of Dodge.

We chose door number three and started the drip. Sitting in the hospital waiting for something to happen was stressful. It's a good thing the U.S. Open golf was on the television in the birthing room. Every so often Jodi would ask me what time it was. I couldn't figure out why until she explained to me that she was having contractions.

Jodi's contractions took a while to get going but when they did, boy oh boy, did things move quickly. From the time she asked for the epidural to the time it took to get an anesthesiologist up to give it most of the dilation

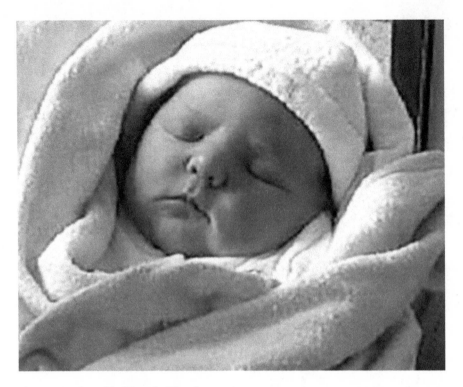

Avery, one day old. (Family Photo)

had occurred. The epidural didn't work and Jodi had to see it through the old-fashioned way. I had to work hard as well. Not passing out from what I was witnessing was my main task.

When it was all said and done our little princess, Avery, was born three weeks less a day early at 5:17 PM and weighing in at a respectable seven pounds seven ounces. Jodi's doctor recovered from her heart attack and Jodi's parents missed Cyndi Lauper but got to see Cher. There was even enough time for my mom to make it to the waiting room where I got to give her a big hug after Avery was born.

All-in-all, it worked out just swimmingly.

That said, two days later I would give Avery her first bath, and when I took the cloth to her head I managed to wipe a big stripe of her peach fuzz hair clean off her head. I was assured this was normal, but the poor girl waited two years before she had enough hair to put into pigtails.

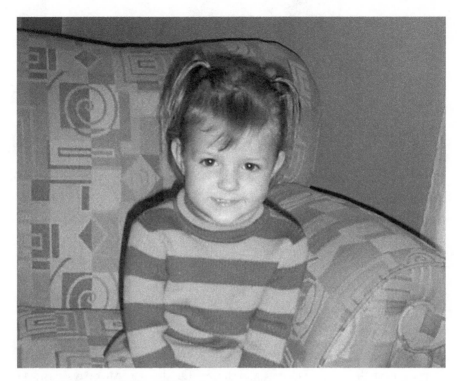

Avery, two years old. (Family Photo)

FROM THE MOUTHS OF BABES

The moments between a child's first breath and their first words are precious. In between the bouts of crying, the sounds babies make are soul-soothing and a baby's laugh is infectious. Once the words start flowing, though, well you'd better watch out because as the saying goes, kids say the darndest things.

Avery was a "talkative" baby. She cooed and giggled and told stories and laughed. Her first words, like most other babies, were "dada" and "mama" (in that order, I should point out). The first word to pass her lips after those, however, was… non-standard.

Avery wasn't yet a year to this world and she was already the center of our universe. This was late 2002 or early 2003 and back in the days of digital cameras that weren't integrated in with every cell phone. They weren't tiny, either, and the resolution was terrible. But, not having to develop film to see your pictures was fantastic.

Avery was up to something cute and Jodi sent me upstairs to get the digital camera from the computer room. I bounded up the stairs and had reached the top step when I heard Jodi yell up to me, "Never mind, she stopped doing it."

Loud enough to be heard downstairs I yelped out, "Shit!" and you guessed it, half a heartbeat later our little potty-mouthed princess parroted dada not once but several times.

"Shit. Shit. Shit? Shit!"

What makes it even more special is she said each one with a different inflection and unique tone. I'm not sure how long it went on but I do remember the look on Jodi's face when I came back downstairs. In my defense, Avery's cousins call that "Grandma's word" (my mother) so I come by it naturally and am at least passing it down properly through the generations.

It wasn't all expletives as Avery grew up, though. There was also human anatomy. We had Avery in swim lessons from the age of three months so she was no stranger to the pool. One day, we were in the change room at the local pool and it was one of those family change rooms where moms with sons and dads with daughters could change and shower. On this particular day every stall is filled with a mom and a son except for me and Avery. I'm getting changed and Avery points to my thing and says, "What's that?" I ignored her and she says again with more force now, "Daddy, what's THAT?"

I lean in close and whisper, "That's daddy's penis."

What happened next? You guessed it. She yelled at the top of her lungs, as only a child can do, *"DADDY HAS A PENIS. I NO HAVE PEANUTS, I HAVE A BUHGINA. DADDY HAS A PENIS!"*

Needless to say the moms in all the other stalls got quite a good laugh out of it and I stayed a few shades of embarrassed for quite some time afterward.

Of course, not everything that's ever come out of Avery's mouth has been body parts and cussing. She's a smart kid and from an early age it was clear that her brain worked more like her mother's than it did mine.

On the way home from the doctor (she had an ear infection) we turned out of the parking lot and she said to me, "Daddy, what street is this?" I said, "It's March Road". "March?" she said. "Where does your birthday live?"

You see, my birthday is in March. Jodi's is in August and Avery's is in

June. When I told her that we were driving on March Road the first thing she thought was, "Hey, this is March Road. Daddy's birthday is in March. Daddy's birthday must live here!" Genius? You tell me. It only took me five minutes to figure out what the heck she was talking about!

Other things Avery has blurted out over the years are less nuanced. I remember one time Jodi was reading Avery one of those *Dora the Explorer* books that help young kids learn to read. It used pictures of common objects in with the text of the book so that when you came to certain words, the picture was there and the kid could point to the picture and learn to associate the word with the thing. For instance, when the story came to a point with a tree in it, there was a picture of a tree with "tree" written under it so the kid could hopefully put two and two together.

Jodi was reading this book with Avery, and it was about baseball or sports or something like that. There was definitely a spot involving baseball because they came to a point in the book where Dora slid into home base and there was a picture of home plate. Jodi said, "...and then Dora slides into home...." and she points to the picture of home base and Avery said, "Depot!" That's my girl.

Avery came by her love of words naturally and Jodi and I read to her every day from a very young age. Some of the words and phrases she uttered, however, didn't always make sense. This is expected from most children, I would think, but this is also an area Jodi and I can take some credit for. It started with a nickname.

Avery Jordan Wilks Butters is the name on her birth certificate, and while simply calling her Avery would have sufficed Jodi and I were determined to have a proper nickname for her. "Peanut" was a first attempt (Peanut Butters, ha!) but didn't take (mostly because it was way too obvious). "AJ" was also tried but the moniker never quite fit her personality. When Avery discovered Disney princesses we knew "Princess" would have staying power. "Princess Avery" didn't have that certain flair though. It needed... more.

Jodi has always had an affinity for using funny rhyming names for people. I was "Andrew Bandrew" and Avery was "Avery Bavery" but "Princess Avery Bavery" also didn't have the right ring to it. At some point something switched. "Avery Bavery" became "Paloney Baloney." We don't know how. It just did. From there the transition to "Princess Paloney Baloney" was inevitable.

That name was too much of a mouthful and eventually we shortened it to simply "Princess P". Now, your guess is as good as mine as to how the next change happened but at some point the "P" became "Pants" and "Princess Pants" was, in the etymological sense, born. Of course, that was eventually shortened down to simply "Pants" and that's what we use in our day-to-day interactions though if we're being casual we'll use "Pantalonies". Don't ask why; we don't have any idea. As you will see, Avery's proper title, "Princess Pants", is still used in formal correspondence.

OH, THE THINGS SHE DOES

In my small number of years as a father I have noticed that the ratio of funny or silly or cute or ridiculous things a child says is directly proportional to those things that they do. Avery was no exception.

Avery was always a good eater. Okay, there was that one time at only two months old that she decided she wouldn't have anything to do with the one bottle I fed her every day to give Jodi a break from breastfeeding, but I'm not counting that as being a bad eater so much as a picky eater. She wasn't a picky eater for very long, though.

One day we left Avery to her own devices on the main floor of our townhome. She couldn't have been two years old at the time so there was only so much damage she could do. I'm not sure what Jodi and I were up to but we gated her in what we thought was a toddler-proofed area and off we went. We weren't gone long, but anyone who has ever seen kids this age in action knows that it doesn't take long. They're like destruction ninjas.

Jodi and I returned to discover that Avery had gotten up onto the dining room table. She was sitting in the middle of it happy as a clam… eating the butter straight from the butter dish. I didn't know whether to discipline her or give her a high-five.

Butter wasn't the only thing Avery was passionate about. From an early age she had a sincere love of shoes. Now, I'm not going to tell you the name of the person from whom she inherited this particular infatuation, but I will give you a hint: it's her mother. At one point Avery had more than twenty pairs of shoes. *Twenty.* For a three-year-old. Anyhow, they say you should choose your battles, and this wasn't one I was prepared to die on the hill for. I did come close once, though.

I woke up one morning and was preparing something for Avery to eat when one of her TV shows ended. Well, because kids' attention spans are about thirty seconds long, the TV folks fill the time with other little creative shows to carry them over to the next episode. Being Television Ontario (kind of like the Ontario Canada version of PBS) there were no commercials. Instead was showing a filler spot called "Twinkle Toes".

It was all about dancing and body movement and so forth. The opening for the show had a large number of pink and blue shoes of various styles moving back and forth across the screen as the show title was written out in some scripted font. Avery was across the room when this show came on and she ran to the television and when all the shoes started moving around she hugged the TV. My daughter hugged a television because it was showing her dancing shoes. At least it wasn't a show about butter.

After the "incident" with having U.S. Open golf on during Avery's birth there was a bit of a moratorium on the sport for a while. That all changed when Jodi and I took Avery to play mini golf one warm Sunday evening. There was a little course not too far from our house. Each hole had an animal on it, and they had a big polar bear out front. Avery loved polar bears at that age and we figured she would have fun.

This was her first mini-golf outing. In fact she had never even held a putter before. I had tried on many occasions to show her how so I could get a feel for if she golfed left or right (so I could buy her the proper clubs) but she wanted nothing to do with it.

We got to the course and the guy at the counter took one look at her and decided she was too small to charge to play. Score! I saved three bucks. We got to the first tee which was some sort of funny tube that was supposed to be a rocket (okay, so not all holes had an animal). I put the ball down on the mat and stood above Avery and showed her how to put her feet and then I asked her to hold the club. She held it left, so we went with that. I held onto her hands to keep the putter straight and told her to pull it back and then "whack the ball."

She did exactly as I instructed and the ball went sailing through the long tube and out the other end. It whipped right past the hole to a railing, where it bounced off and took a few little hops before landing right in the cup. A hole-in-one on her first ever shot with a golf club. Avery was already having a blast but kept calling the game "Mickey Mouse" instead of "mini golf" and she didn't have a clue what a "putter" or "club" was. To her it was a "hockey stick" or "whacker thing".

Avery cruised along until about the eighth hole. Right before she "teed off" she looked down and saw a whole bunch of little caterpillars on the Astroturf. She dropped her putter and screamed, "Caterpillars! Look, little caterpillars! They will turn into butterflies. This one is away from his mommy and daddy," then she picked it up and walked it over to another one lying on the ground. "There you go, back home now." Suffice it to say that Avery's game suffered greatly after the discovery of actual wildlife on the course.

We eventually made it to the end of the course. The final hole was a big ramp with a horribly drawn picture of a clown face at the end with a wide open mouth with a hole in it where the ball goes through. Avery said, "What this hole? I have to hit it through the big scary thing?" I had never thought about it but I guess to a kid clowns are scary. This thing was certainly nothing to look at, that's for sure. She hit the ball a few dozen times then crawled up under the protective grate (so the ball doesn't launch into the parking lot) and threw the ball into the hole. She then crawled out and ran around to the other side where she realized for the first time that the ball is not coming back.

Ever.

Of course, this led to a total and complete meltdown as we tried to explain to her that that's how mini golf works. You don't get to keep the ball after the last hole. You have to give it back so someone else can have a turn. In hindsight we probably could have prepared her for that a little better. Oh well, we were still new to all that parenting stuff and sometimes you don't get a hole-in-one.

About eighteen months later Avery brought together her love of shoes with her love of sports and got her first pair of soccer cleats. Her initial foray into the "beautiful game" came the summer after she started junior kindergarten. Avery loved to run around and she definitely loved to kick a ball around, but putting the two together didn't quite have the same allure.

I should mention that when she started playing soccer she was wearing glasses that had translucent tape over one of the lenses. She needed one eye to work a little harder than the other one so this allowed her to see fuzzy blobs out of the one eye and clearly out of the other one. It also had the unfortunate side effect of diminishing her depth perception. I won't try to embarrass her too much but let's just say she took more than one ball to the face.

During Avery's introductory season I sat on the grass with the other parents and watched every practice and game. In around the third or fourth game of the season many of the kids were starting to get the hang of it. I'm sure the others enjoyed running around and chasing the ball.

The kids played on a quarter field whose long side of the rectangle was the width of a standard soccer pitch. At each end was a small semi-circular net. There were no goalies. There were no offside rules. No positional play at all, come to think of it. There were three things that could happen with that ball:

1) It could go out of bounds.

2) It could go into the net to count as a goal.

3) It could get booted around by one big swarm of four and five year olds.

You can probably guess that items #1 and #3 happened a lot.

This one particular game there was quite a lot of swarming going on and not much else. It was the most frustrating thing to watch because nothing happened. Most of the time you couldn't even make out your kid in the swarm. Well, Avery must have lost interest because I couldn't see her in the swarm. Sitting on the ground was comfortable, but not great for seeing anything down the other end of the field.

Then, I heard the chuckles coming from the other parents. The swarm moved off to the side and there was Avery, way down the other end of the field running around the net with her arms outstretched pretending to be an airplane. All the other parents looked over at me. I said, "She's providing air cover," and went back to cheering.

SHE COMES BY IT NATURALLY

Between the two of us growing up, Jodi and I managed to keep the Emergency Departments at local hospitals busy. Whether it was a finger or an arm or a leg or even a head, you could count on at least one broken something every year. So, from the second Avery could walk, Jodi and I have been on tenterhooks waiting for it to happen to her. Well, on her first day of junior kindergarten it almost happened.

Avery was four years old and it was a warm September afternoon. Avery's three-and-a-half-month-old baby brother was in the stroller and Jodi was taking her to school. Not a few days earlier Avery had received her first pair of glasses. From the beginning she had to have tape on the one lens to strengthen her other eye. It didn't bother her at all but as you heard about during her soccer days it made for some interesting moments.

On this particular day, Avery was excited to be at school and having new experiences and meeting friends and playing on the playground. It turns out she was not alone in her excitement, and there were other kids running around and generally unaware of anyone else while at the same time trying to soak in everything around them.

As luck would have it, Avery and this other kid were running full tilt around the same corner in opposite directions and, BAM!, they collided. Thankfully, and at least partially due to the fact that kids are mostly bouncy until the age of ten and their combined weight was less than a hundred pounds, there were no cracked skulls or broken bones. What did happen was Avery broke her glasses and ended up with a nice cut above her eye. She survived, and afterward proudly sported her scar from her big collision.

Only a couple of short years later it was time to put a helmet on her and teach her to ride a bike. Naturally, I was going to record this moment for posterity so Jodi won the job of holding the seat and running behind Avery until she either fell over or figured it out.

It had already been a long morning of running back and forth (for Jodi) while I stood in the sunshine and recorded video after video of failure. Not to be deterred, the team of mom and daughter persisted until real progress started to occur. With tensions running high and Jodi running behind the bike, it looked like riding was imminent. Camera at the ready and with the sun casting long shadows on our quiet suburban side street, Jodi ran with her hand on the back of the seat and then let go.

Avery hadn't peddled for a count of one Mississippi before Jodi took one look at her trajectory and started shouting, "Not into the car! Not into the car!"

Two Mississippi counts later it was clear that pedaling wasn't the problem but steering and/or stopping was. On the fourth Mississippi the speed wobble took over and launched both bike and rider at the front bumper of the neighbour's car. After the telltale sound of a bike hitting pavement Avery let out an, "Ow!" and I stopped recording.

There were tears.

In a move that surprised no one, daddy was ordered to cease the recording of all bike riding activities. But still, Avery persisted, and within fifteen minutes was proudly pedaling on her own, and steering and braking all by herself. As for the neighbour's car, it was fine. As for the crash video, it was on YouTube within an hour: https://youtu.be/TK6T_pMDugs

HERO IN THE MAKING

It didn't take long for Avery to go from being indestructible to indispensable. Avery was an active kid right from the get-go and as you've read was no stranger to bumps and bruises and falling (lots of falling). It was just a kid being a kid, though. As her paediatrician told me at her second year checkup, "Bumps and bruises on kids are a good thing. It means they're active. I get worried when I don't see them." None of Avery's wipeouts were due to a lack of attentiveness.

In fact, Avery has always been an observant as well as compassionate girl. This is never more apparent than when you saw her interact with her little brother. With three years and eleven months difference between the two, Jodi and I were concerned that they would not grow close, but not only did Avery love spending time with her little brother, she cared for him a great deal.

When AJ was two years old and Avery was six, we found out the hard way that AJ was allergic to peanuts. This was a terrifying shock for mom and dad, and a real blow to Avery's steady march towards independence, as she had learned that if she was hungry she could make herself a peanut butter sandwich.

With the peanut allergy as severe as it was, we eliminated anything in the house to do with peanuts. Avery was devastated, but understood why and never complained, and she never made AJ feel like he was missing out on anything and life went on.

Fast forward four years, when AJ had assumed the role of the six-year-old and Avery was ten going on twenty-five. It was shortly after the most anxiety-riddled holiday of the year: Halloween. As per household procedures, Jodi and I had both independently vetted all the candy before putting each of the kid's hauls into zipper close freezer bags with their names written on the outside in permanent marker.

Jodi and I were on the couch after supper and watching something on the television. AJ asked if he could have something from his treat bag. Of course, we said he could and he sat down at the table to pick something out. He had no sooner taken a bite when Avery happened by and picked up the wrapper to see what he was eating.

"Mommy, daddy," she said, "there's peanuts in this!"

"Can't be. Nothing in his bag has the 'May contain peanuts' warning."

Avery brought the wrapper over to me and pointed to the ingredients list.

"Peanuts are the third ingredient," she said.

I jumped up off the couch and ordered AJ to spit out what was in his mouth. Then, I took him to the bathroom and made him wash his mouth out with water and told him not to swallow anything. Then, we brushed his teeth and gargled with mouthwash followed by another rinse and spit with water. Then, we sat him down on the couch, Epi Pens at the ready and we waited.

Twenty minutes passed and he didn't have any hives and there was no swelling anywhere to his face or throat. We thought we were in the clear. Then, he projectile vomited across the living room. At this point I wasn't sure if it was just the anxiety that did it or if it was a reaction to him swallowing any of that chocolate bar, but off to the hospital he went. They kept an eye on him and pumped him full of Benadryl and after a couple hours they let us go home.

Candy was re-inspected and household procedures were updated to include the reading of every ingredient and not counting on the "may contain" warnings. Every year since then I checked the label on that chocolate bar to see if they added the warning or if peanuts appeared only in the ingredients list. I'm happy to report that after four years the label now contains a warning.

That was the beginning of our daughter's career as a superhero. The rest would unfold just a couple years later when a mole on AJ's neck would start us down the path of discovering Avery's scoliosis and eventually solidify Avery's place as the person admired most in the entire world.

At this point you might be asking, "I beg your pardon? How does one get from a mole on your son's neck to your daughter's scoliosis diagnosis?" and that would be a perfectly legitimate question. One that is best answered by Jodi's first family scoliosis journey blog entry.

JODI: AND IT STARTED LIKE THIS

Monday, September 29, 2014 (113 Days to Surgery)

I have been looking for more 'real' information about this whole scoliosis diagnosis and surgery and what—what happens, how she will feel—and I haven't found it—though maybe I am using Google incorrectly and that is why. So I decided we, as a family, could maybe share our thoughts as we move forward through this journey, and hopefully through a smooth and uneventful recovery—but then if there is someone else one day asking these same questions, they can stumble upon this and have at least one family's perspective on things.

(Oh, and we are Canadian, so this surgery is covered by our universal healthcare system—but I will still complain a little about wait times.)

So the story to now: I (Mom here) am not a big taker of the kids to the doctor. We go for shots as needed, and of course as babies I had them in for all their check-ups, but now that they are older, doctor's visits (outside of the immunization schedule) are for specific complaints that can't be otherwise treated. So back in March 2014 I noticed that my little Dude had a mole on his neck that he kept scratching at—so just to be safe, I took him in to have it checked. On being brought back to the exam room, the nurse casually asked when I was last in with the Dude. I replied that it had probably been a year and a half, maybe two years? Her reply was, "Almost three." So when the doctor came in, I asked if I should be scheduling something for Avery as I figured it had been likely the same amount of time, to which her reply was

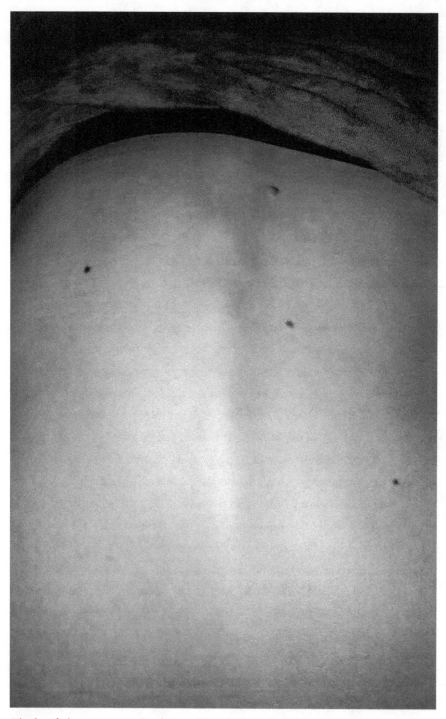

The bend that sent us to the doctor. (Family Photo)

something like, "No, we don't really need her to come in annually if there is nothing wrong, but the one thing I would look for in an otherwise healthy eleven-year-old would be if her spine was straight, but you can do that easily enough at home. Just have her stand up and bend over to touch her toes and look. You'll see. :)" And yes, I believe there was a smiley in that sentence.

So half-jokingly I did just that, and this is what I saw: (see photo at left).

So I called the doctor's office and made an appointment. We saw the doctor the next week (and on arrival, the doctor said she thought I may have been joking to have scheduled this appointment—in a nice way). She took a quick look and immediately referred us to Avery's paediatrician from when she was maybe one-and-a-half years old. That appointment happened a few days later—at the end of March.

I hated the paediatrician appointment—she asked me four times if I was sure I hadn't noticed this before now—which offended me; though it was suggested to me afterwards that what she was trying to get at was how quickly this had developed. Had I noticed it last year, but not thought much of it, or did it just show up with no warning? I felt like the—worst—Mom—ever. She sent us immediately across to the hospital for scoliosis screen x-rays and worked up a referral to a paediatric orthopaedic surgeon in Hamilton. Those x-rays suggested a 43 degree curve.

The specialist appointment was scheduled for early May 2014—and last minute I had a work function to attend, so I sent Avery with her Dad (who is an awesome dad and totally capable to do this appointment—in fact probably more so that me.) I mean— we figured she would maybe get a brace, maybe physio, maybe chiropractic. We were not at all expecting to come away from that appointment with a surgery is the only option diagnosis. The curve, when corrected with a 1 cm piece of wood, was presenting as an "S" with 47 degree curve at the top and 50ish at the bottom—but the point being, once the curve is over 45 (at most 40 by many people's opinions), bracing would only make it worse, so surgery becomes the only option. I thought I felt like the—worst—Mom—ever at the paediatricians. Not being there for this appointment made me feel like the—absolute—worst—Mom—ever and really by the time they were done, it was nearly noon—but

I basically missed any worthwhile content at the session I was at because I kept getting hit with waves of awful.

So we absorb surgery. We talk about what this means—Andrew was told that once the surgery is scheduled, we should plan on having Avery bank her blood so that she can be give her own blood if any is needed during surgery. We were told that the surgery would take approximately ten hours, and then Avery would need to be in the ICU for a day. Following that, she would be in the hospital for one week. Then home, but off school for three more weeks, then gradually returning to school, with the plan that she be back full-time within four months of her surgery. FOUR MONTHS?!?! Oh, and no physical activity for about a year.

The follow-up appointment with the surgeon was scheduled for July 2014. This time I went. I will not be missing another appointment—at least not for something work-related. I was under the misguided belief that this appointment would schedule surgery. Avery had updated x-rays taken and the surgeon evaluated them and it seemed that both curves had gotten worse. He does say that his margin of error is 5%, so possibly not, but I was pretty sure that curve looked worse, but what do I know, I am an HR manager. (I swear he said 51 and 57, but Andrew swears I am mistaken). And all we left with was a follow-up appointment in three months and a prescription for physiotherapy and an inversion table (or as the Dude calls it, a diversion table—which I partly think is accurate as that prescription came when I tried to push about timing for surgery.)

So here we are in (almost) October 2014. Our second follow-up appointment was just pushed back to late October from early October and we don't yet have a surgery date. This was Avery last Friday: (see photo at right).

So maybe it is just the way I took the photo, but I feel like there is a visible difference, and not for the better.

Now, I get that there are kids with way worse cases than this. I am super thankful that to this point she hasn't experienced much pain or discomfort and that this diagnosis hasn't limited her ability to do anything. I mean, she just finished playing beach volleyball all summer and field hockey at school. She is doing her physio exercises fairly consistently and practices yoga with her dad once a week.

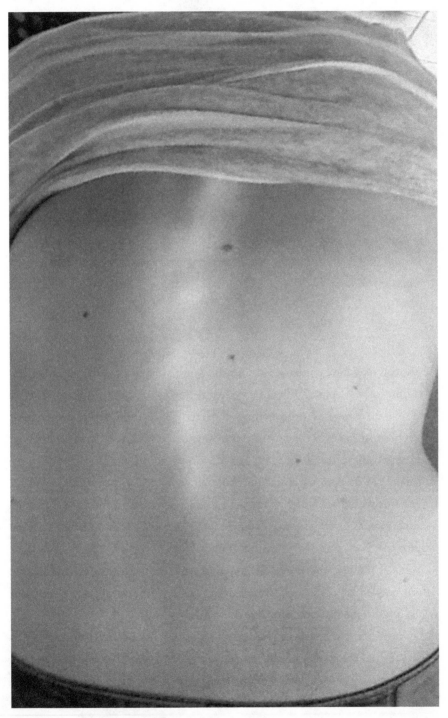

Six months after diagnosis. (Family Photo)

I was told to find her an osteopath by my massage therapist. Another RMT friend suggested I need to find a chiropractor who does something with the 'functional chain' (which I think is a kinesiology thing). I am pretty resigned to surgery, I mean I am all for holistic stuff, and will try lots of stuff to help, but I don't think I am going to find some magic bullet that will bring her up to closer to straight. Oh, and on that subject, our surgeon sent us to this website for information: http://spinal-deformity-surgeon.com/ and I was a little surprised that the correction was to about a 20 degree curve even with the surgery. So, we aren't likely to get Avery completely straight.

Ok, that is enough for the first post. I have invited both Avery (who is affectionately known around here as Princess Pants) and Andrew to post to this blog as well. I mean, you never know what we may learn from one another this way.

—Mom

As you may have gathered from reading Jodi's blog post, scoliosis is a lateral curvature of the spine. When viewed directly from behind, the spine looks bent, like the letter "C" or sometimes the letter "S", but the actual deformity is much more complex. It occurs in three dimensions and Avery's spine was bent and twisted like a spiral staircase. Left uncorrected, the condition would have impacted her internal organs, squeezing them into places they were not meant to be. This would have had an impact on digestion and breathing as her spine became increasingly deformed, squishing her torso like an accordion. There would have been pain—a whole lot of pain.

One of the first questions I get asked is, what caused it? The answer is easy: I don't know. No one knows, not even the doctors. "Idiopathic," they said. This is just a fancy medical term for "we don't know".

Remember that anecdote about Avery crashing her bike? One possible scenario was that she took a tumble on the playground or off her bike and got her spine a little bit out of whack. Something that, had it happened to an adult, would have had them calling their chiropractor the next day. But, because kids are kids and generally pretty bouncy and malleable, Avery thought nothing of it and continued on, at which point she hit a growth spurt which sent her spine off in the wrong direction. This theory aligns pretty will with some known facts about Avery. First, she's clumsy as all get-out. Always has been. Secondly, she grew more than 3.5 inches in the year leading up to her diagnosis.

The next question that usually follows was, "How did they fix it?" That answer was more complicated as it depended on the severity of the curve, location of the deformity relative to her tailbone and neck, age of the child, and so on. In Avery's case, they used metal rods fixed to her spine with screws to straighten her out.

That was the point where people started to turn a little pale and it usually kicked off a flurry of nervous follow-up questions.

Here are the most popular ones:

- *How was it diagnosed?*
- *How long did she have to wait for surgery?*
- *How long was the surgery?*
- *Was Avery scared?*
- *Were you scared?*
- *What exactly did they do to fix it?*
- *How long does it take to heal?*
- *Will she be able to do everything she did before?*
- *Will they take the rods out?*
- *Will she beep when she goes through airport security?*

I suggested that my daughter start journaling her experiences and thoughts in an effort to help her process everything that was being thrown at her. Her mother and my wife, Jodi, immediately went looking on the internet for other people's experiences and didn't come up with anything she found particularly useful. There was a lot of medical information, most of it from the United States (we are in Canada), and a whack of case studies, but very little in terms of what the patient or a parent would experience. So, my genius wife (ever the problem solver), started a blog where we could all contribute and share our perspectives on this life-changing event.

The answer to the most common first question, "How was it diagnosed?" was answered in her first post and as you read, there was a lot of history packed in there. Jodi did an excellent job summarizing what happened between Avery's diagnoses on March 31st to that blog post in late September.

However, there is a lot more to that story. Much like a musical composition, a lot happens in the silence between the notes. We had six months between the diagnosis and the start of the family blog where so much happened while we were, well, waiting for other stuff to happen. But, as with most things, it is best if we start at the beginning.

ONE

THE BEGINNING

I'm in the fortunate position of working in the medical imaging software industry. As such, I am familiar with a variety of medical images that are taken for any number of reasons. I've looked at nuclear medicine scans of glands, PET CT scans designed to find cancer, mammography images in both 2D and 3D, and yes, spinal x-rays.

Medical images are only part of the equation, though. Unless you're a trained medical professional, in this case a radiologist, you'll need the doctor's report to accompany the pictures to make any sense of it. Even then, there are a lot of medical terms that can be terrifying to the untrained eye. That's one of the reasons they don't generally hand a CD of images and doctor's reports to patients and parents. The information contained therein is almost always relayed to the patient by way of a medical professional.

Avery's doctor, our family physician, referred us to a paediatrician who ordered the x-rays, received the images and the report, and then referred Avery to a paediatric orthopaedic surgeon. As there are only a handful of doctors in Ontario who can provide the specialized level of care required, Avery's referral was a 45-minute drive from our house. While not ideal, this was far from a major inconvenience for me and my wife. What benefit this did give us was we were handed a CD of images and the doctor's reports to take with us to the surgeon. It turns out that this is a much more efficient and reliable way to get information

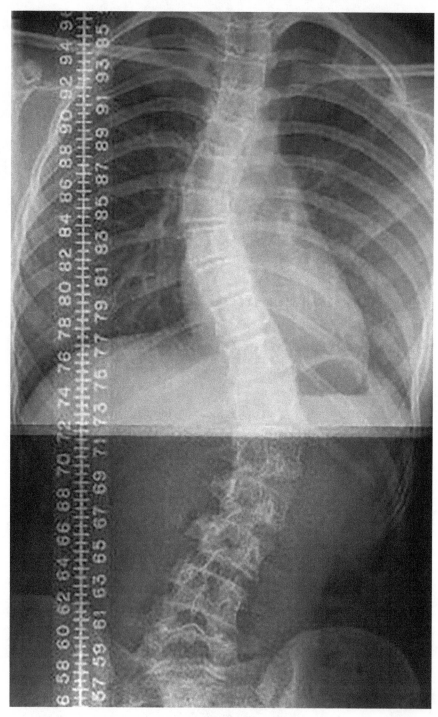

Initial x-rays. March 31, 2014. (Personal Medical Record)

from one medical organization to another. It also meant that I could take a look at what was on the CD and read the report.

Firing up my work computer and popping in the disk, I jumped straight to the images and saw this: *(See X-ray photo at left)*.

Yikes! That is *not* a straight spine. Not even close. That looks scary, but what about the report?

DOCTOR'S REPORT

March 31, 2014 (296 Days to Surgery)

Scoliosis

There is an S type thoracolumbar scoliosis with convexity to the right in the thoracic spine into the left in the lumbar spine. It is centered at T7/ eight in the thoracic spine and T12/L1 in the lumbar spine.

Cobb angle between T5/6 and T 11/12 is 31 degrees and Cobb angle between T11/12 and L 3/4 is 43 degrees.

There is left lateral offset by 3.7 cm.

No underlying congenital vertebral body abnormality is seen.

As you can see, that's not any more reassuring. I had to read it again. Then I read it a third time with a medical dictionary on hand to help with some of the terms. The important pieces of information to extract from this are: a) there were no congenital abnormalities (I had to focus on the fact that of all the terrible things that can happen to a child, ours was dealt a problem that could be fixed), b) there are two curves—one to the right and one to the left—creating the "S" shape, and c) the angles of those curves are 31 and 43 degrees with 0 degrees being perfectly straight. The "T" and "L" letters represent the part of the spine affected.

Avery's "S" curve impacted a lot of vertebrae and the angles were well off of ideal, but what did it all mean? Armed with this information and five or six weeks before the appointment with the surgeon it meant a lot of frustrated waiting.

One of the first things we did was get Avery and me into yoga. I had been saying for months that I should start going and this was the catalyst that would do it. Jodi looked up some local yoga studios and one of them had a bunch of referrals and testimonials on it. Jodi noticed that the first referral on the page was from our family doctor and a few minutes later Avery and I were signed up for "Breathe Into Motion—Level 1" yoga with Mike Chapman.

Mike's yoga system starts at Level 1 and is built on weeks and weeks of fundamentals geared toward people who are rehabilitating injuries. It was perfect for an out-of-shape dad with a bad back, and Avery, who just needed to stay flexible and increase her strength. Several weeks of introductory yoga passed and the appointment with the surgeon was upon us.

THE FIRST APPOINTMENT
May 9, 2015 (256 days to surgery)

At the last minute, Jodi had to attend a work function in the city so I was flying solo for the first appointment. Up to this point I had been fortunate to have Jodi beside me for all the big stuff (and a ton of the little stuff, too). She is also the brains of the operation, so suffice it to say I was nervous. First up were a ton of x-rays. The surgical resident ordered the wrong ones at first, and then he identified a difference in length of Avery's legs so she had to go back for a third set, this time with a block of wood to put under one foot. Even though I know the radiation dose is very small, especially for a modern digital x-ray machine, I have to admit, I joked that if she had any more scans done, she'd glow in the dark.

When we finally got to speak to the surgeon directly he sat down, pulled up one of Avery's x-rays, described in plain terms what was going on with her spine, told us the angles of the curves—I don't remember what they were exactly but they were both worse than the original doctor's report—and then said eight words which knocked the wind out of both Avery and me:

"Avery's only option at this point is surgery."

Avery went into shock, with her innocent eyes as big as pie plates and filled with panic. There was a tremble in her bottom lip and she sat motionless in the chair. I clenched my teeth and looked into the doctor's eyes in an attempt to keep it together. On the inside I felt like I was going to be sick. The surgeon said that there was a five degree margin of error on each of the measurements, but even if he factored that in she was dangerously close to "the point of no

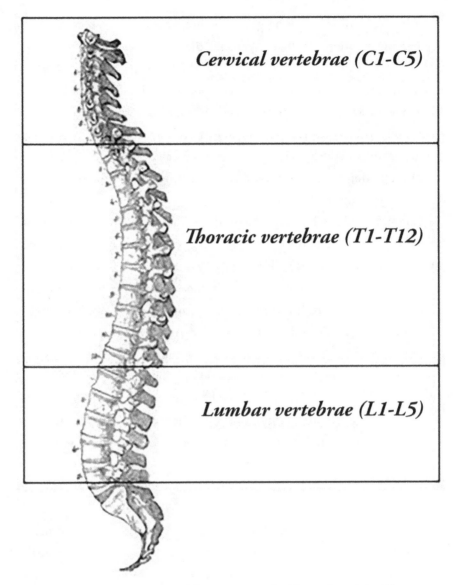

Cervical vertebrae (C1-C5)

Thoracic vertebrae (T1-T12)

Lumbar vertebrae (L1-L5)

The Human Spine. (Anatomy of the Human Body, Henry Gray (1918))
Overlay by Andrew F. Butters

return", if not past it already. This point was critical. It meant that if left unchecked Avery's spine would continue to deteriorate. The only question left in the surgeon's mind at this point was how fast it would deteriorate. We set a follow up appointment for two months later and headed down to the car.

It wasn't until the parking garage before we got in the car that Avery showed any emotion. Before she got into the car I gave her a hug and told her that everything was going to be okay. She cried in my arms for several minutes. I don't even remember at what point I told Jodi, whether it was via text while we were still upstairs or whether I called her from the car or when I got home. All I know is it felt like one of those scenes in a movie where a bomb goes off and the hero is wandering around all disoriented and confused with his ears ringing. Only in this case I wasn't the hero. Heck, there was no hero. At least not yet.

I am sure I didn't ask enough questions. If I had to do it over again I would have researched more of the options available, prepared myself for surgery as a possible solution, and had a list of questions to ask.

I'm also sure I wasn't the best father in those moments after we heard the memorable eight words. If I had to do it over again I would not have left her side. There was a moment where I was speaking to the surgeon in the hall and Avery was alone in the exam room. I didn't want her to hear the questions I was asking. They terrified me and I could only imagine how terrified they would make her, and I didn't want to send her into a panic any more than she already was. I suppose that's forgivable given she was only eleven at the time and I was trying to protect her. Still, it took me too long to give her a hug. That part I regret every day.

I told her that she didn't have to go to school when we got back and that if she wanted to go home and talk about it that it was perfectly okay. She decided to go to school. I think this was good for her as it allowed her to process the information in a setting in which she was familiar and where she felt safe. There was no one else at home and it would have just been the two of us moping around until Jodi got back from Toronto. Besides, a gaggle of eleven and twelve year old girls would probably have a better sense of how to console Avery than I would. I called my mother and cried.

Jodi and I talked about what it meant for the surgery. We needed to get a second opinion, which we had to set up through Avery's surgeon. We felt it strange that we had to go through our surgeon to get a second opinion but it made sense considering there are so few doctors in the province that have the skill-set and experience required. I'm better at the tactical stuff so I was tasked with communicating with the various administrative staff to square away appointments and things of that nature. What I am not, however, is blessed with an abundance of patience and with two months until the next appointment I was going to need every bit I could muster. With patience in short supply, waiting wasn't exactly my forte, and I was about to do what felt like a lifetime of it.

TWO

WAITING

While two months between appointments seemed like a long time, I figured the experienced surgeon knew what he was doing. That didn't make it any easier on me, though. Naturally impatient, I needed to focus on something, and as luck would have it yoga was that something. Yoga Mike was being his usual amazing self. For ninety minutes each week he would instruct Avery on aspects of posture and alignment and even gave her a few exercises designed to help with her scoliosis. There was a brief moment where Avery's hopes were artificially raised when she read that Mike had worked with a girl to reverse her scoliosis, but her case was not nearly as severe as Avery's. Still, these things would help, and Avery's surgeon and surgical resident were in agreement with Mike on that front, so we went to our Level 1 classes every week.

The week following our first appointment I called Dr. Missiuna's office to get a referral set up.

The instructions were as follows:

1) ask Dr. Missiuna to identify a suitable doctor to provide the second opinion,

2) request Dr. Missiuna's office contact said doctor to set up the second opinion, and

3) wait.

I followed these instructions to the letter. Dr. Missiuna recommended Dr. Zeller at Toronto's Sick Kids hospital. Not too shabby considering it's one of the country's leading children's facilities.

Two weeks passed.

Nothing.

Three weeks passed.

Nothing.

After a month, I called the office again asking for something, anything, to let me know what was going on. The office assistant's response when asked if there was any word on Avery's second opinion didn't exactly fill me with confidence.

"Oh, you wanted the second opinion? I thought you were still thinking about it."

Seriously? It took every bit of patience I could muster to not completely lose my cool. Do you want to know what the really good part of all this was? All she had to do was fill out a form online and provide me with the referral confirmation number.

With the second appointment right around the corner I made a note of the performance, or lack thereof, of the administrative assistant as well as all the questions I could think of. Dr. Missiuna said that there were no bad questions and that we should all write them down as soon as we thought of them. In the nine weeks between appointments I managed to write down a page of them using every other line as well as inside the margin.

The days leading up to the second appointment were long, but I kept going to yoga with Avery and tried to stay positive. Again, I tried to focus on the fact that this was something that was fixable. Jodi was with us this time and it would be the first time she met Dr. Missiuna. There were more x-rays and lots of sitting around waiting. The only thing that was on my mind was her angles. By looking at Avery you wouldn't have noticed a difference, but that's what all the fancy equipment and expert doctor were for.

As it happened, that was the only thing that the doctor was concerned with as well. Avery got lit up like an x-ray Christmas tree again and the good doctor did his measuring. I was a little disappointed he wasn't using the software my company makes, but I'm sure it did the job. What he found was that Avery's angles were five degrees worse. With a five-degree margin of error that meant that Avery's best case scenario was that her curves were stable. However, looking at the pictures side-by-side you could easily see that they were worse.

There was no turning back.

This was a bit of a gut punch for everybody. Dr. Missiuna explained the point of no return. Avery's spine would never straighten on its own and if she wore a brace it would just squeeze her in the wrong direction. This was where we learned the true severity of her condition. Gravity was her enemy at this point and left unchecked her spine would collapse.

Still, Avery's situation was not dire. She was on the list for surgery even though we had no sense of where on the list. All the doctor would say was that if he was lucky, he got an operating room suitable for this type of surgery once a month. Seeing as we were in July and the doctor was taking all of December off, the likelihood of surgery in 2015 was small. Spring of 2015 was more of a possibility, with the surgery happening sooner if her condition worsened.

Having to endure more than six months of waiting was going to drive me insane. Naturally, I had concerns about the toll this was going to have on Avery as well. There had to be something we could do. Jodi asked that very question and both Dr. Missiuna and his resident felt that continuing with yoga was a great idea. He also prescribed some physiotherapy and continued use of the "diversion table."

—

The summer passed quickly, as summers have a tendency to do, but I didn't miss a yoga class with Avery. If we couldn't make it on one day we'd make up the class on another day that week. With so much uncertainty and anxiety weighing over her I wanted to make sure there was at least one thing that was consistent. The hardest part for me was the waiting. As I've said, I'm not a patient man, and I had to resist the urge to call and ask about the second opinion referral every day. I had the next appointment booked on the calendar, October 6—which later got pushed out to October 20—and I'd be lying if I said I didn't have a desk calendar with a little countdown.

September arrived and with it seventh grade, and it was almost a certainty that Avery would have surgery at some point before the end of the school year. Jodi and I went to the school and talked with her home room French and English teachers, the principal, and the vice principal, and the gym teachers (pretty much every adult Avery would come into contact with). I knew Avery was a good student but that didn't stop me from worrying about how much time she was going to miss. Thankfully, it wasn't eighth grade or high school where the impact of so much time away was much greater.

Everyone at the school understood Avery's situation and were eager to do anything they could to accommodate her needs. There were lots of questions, the two most common being, "When will you know?" and "How long will Avery be away from school?"

Answering the first question with any specifics wasn't possible so I always went with the standard, "Sometime this school year." Answering the second was easier because it was more of a known quantity. Though, in the mind of a twelve-year-old, the concept of spending months away from all your friends and missing out on schoolwork could be a hard one to come to terms with. Thankfully, Jodi had the blog up and running within a few weeks of school starting and Jodi and I, and especially Avery, had an outlet to share her thoughts. Which brings us to the start of the blog and hearing from Avery for the first time.

AVERY: MY SIDE OF THE STORY

October 2, 2014 (110 days to surgery)

It all started when my brother kept itching at a mole. He was itching at it so often that mom decided to take him to the doctors. I didn't go with them so I don't know what happened, but when they got home mom asked me to bend over and touch my toes. I couldn't touch my toes but she got what she wanted, to see my back. And what did she see? A big fat curve.

Up Until Now

So this is what happened from when we found out to right now on October 2nd.

You already heard the story from my mom but here it is from me. So my mom comes home from the doctors with my brother and asks me to bend over and touch my toes so she can check for scoliosis. I couldn't touch my toes but I was still bent over enough for her to see the BIG CURVE in my spine. I'm still bent over and she's calling my dad over to see it, just to make sure she's not imagining it. And what do you know? She's not. I have scoliosis (BTW SCOLIOSIS SUCKS!). So, now you know my side of the beginning. My mom has already told the rest so I don't need to tell you again. But here's a tip, one of the things I've been thinking every so often now is "I can't do it anymore, I just can't. I wish I didn't have to worry about this anymore. I wish I never had to worry about this!" And yes, I bet every one with scoliosis wishes they never got it, but really there's nothing you can do about it except have the surgery. So, I deal with it and remind myself that after the surgery I'm going to be five foot seven! But that's only my way of coping with it. Find your own way to make it not so bad and DON'T LET IT GET TO YOU!

—Princess Pants

JODI: WAIT TIMES SUCK

October 3, 2014 (109 Days to Surgery)

I am really lucky at my work. I have been assured by my boss and the President that they will support me to take whatever time I may need to get through all of this, and that if there is one thing not to worry about it is work. But here's the thing—I totally do worry. At this point in time I am hopeful (or anxious) that the surgery will take place in February 2015. It is entirely possible my place of work will be gearing up for what could be a massive strike right around that time (and I happen to be the Director of HR responsible for managing our labour relations portfolio). Oh, and one of my team may also need to be off for totally legitimate reasons of her own—at a schedule that is also somewhat out of her control. And I mean we are planning and speaking of contingencies, but none of those options are as good as me being there.

So I worry. And complain that I can't seem to get a date or even a closer estimate of a date. And to be fair, I haven't made one phone call about any of this—I leave that to Andrew who is way more reliable and self-contained that I am. But seriously! The Paediatric Canadian Access Targets for Surgery (P-CATS) List suggests that assuming her scoliosis was "stable" she should have had surgery within six months of diagnosis, but here we are six months later and we still don't have a date. And I don't think it is stable. But I am not a doctor.

Our next appointment with the surgeon was just rescheduled (by snail mail in a letter addressed to my daughter!) for two weeks later. And I know, it is only two weeks, and I chose to believe that it is for some legitimate reason, but still—who doesn't use a phone or at least email?

And I don't think I shared that when I asked the surgeon about getting this scheduled at our last appointment, his reply was that he is only permitted to do this particular surgery once per month—so that is quite limiting. Apparently it is a big and costly surgery, so even though there are people needing it, the paediatric hospital we are dealing with prefers the less costly, less time consuming ones. Oh—and we were referred in FREAKING MAY for a second opinion appointment at the leading paediatric hospital in the country and have yet to have that appointment booked either. So yay! Free health care, unless you really need it, otherwise get in line and maybe we'll get to you in a few months.

I just want a date. I mean is there a reason we can't get booked for February with a one-month move possibility? Even that would be better than this.

But I will push it again on October 20.

And lastly—donate blood if you can. My little girl may need it, and if not mine, someone else's. I can't—the risk of me being a walking mad-cow incubator still exists, and it seems cannot be confirmed (or denied) officially without a biopsy of my dead brain—see, you travel the world when you are young, and these are the consequences.

—Mom

ANDREW: OVERLY EMOTIONAL
HYPOCHONDRIAC FATHER WEIGHS IN

October 4, 2014 (108 Days to Surgery)

So my wife and daughter have weighed in so it's my turn to share some thoughts. Jodi mentioned a couple times that if she was incorrect about something I'd jump in and correct her. That won't be necessary as she got the important stuff right.

Having to absorb the news during that first appointment was pretty tough. Between Jodi and me it's clear I'm the overly emotional one, and I wanted so much to hold it together and keep Avery thinking positively that I'm afraid I may have swung the pendulum the other direction afterwards and in the car on the way home. Was I not compassionate enough? Did I hide too much of what I was feeling? Questions that will never be answered that bother me. All I know at this point is that I'm super proud of our little girl. Have you read her post? It was her first ever blog post and it was about her having to have spinal surgery. Talk about a challenge! I think my first ever blog post was about how I get frustrated with people screwing up my fast food order.

It's been a long, frustrating year since May. On one hand I have every confidence in Avery's surgeon and all of the staff at the hospital. On the other we have the waiting, and the waiting, and the waiting. Have I mentioned the waiting? I see that Jodi just did a post that talked about the waiting. I don't think it can be overstated how frustrating it is. Now that being said, the big trade off of all this not costing us anything is the waiting. They can only do one surgery a month at the hospital and there are a lot of kids on that list, so we wait our turn. We get Avery checked every few months and when the tables turn she gets bumped higher up on the list. It's not a perfect system (don't even get me started on the second opinion we're still waiting for—and have been since the summer), but it's the one we have. Play the cards you're dealt, I suppose.

So how's the overly emotional hypochondriac father doing? Not bad. I work for a medical imaging software company so I have access to all sorts of pre- and post-op scans from just about every medical procedure you can think of, including spinal surgeries. Pro tip: don't look at them. We *don't get the story behind any of the images. They're all anonymous and are mixed in with different reports and a good many of them are extreme cases. Let's just say flipping through a database of random test data is the shortest path to a panic attack.*

I did manage to find images of a girl whose spine angles were similar to Avery's. I'm not sure how Avery or Jodi feel about it, but for me it's comforting to see what they can do and how it works out. It's also reassuring to know that this is a well-established procedure and that Avery's surgeon has done more than a few. So there's that.

For now we go to yoga every Wednesday (big shout out to Mike at Breathe Into Motion Yoga Studios who has been amazing with Avery) and we wait (and wait and wait) for her follow up appointment on October 20, and as Princess Pants so eloquently put it, find our own way to make it not so bad.

—Dad

JODI: SECOND OPINION
October 15, 2014 (97 Days to Surgery)

Yay! After five months of waiting, there was a letter addressed to the "parent or guardian of" from Sick Kids for the second opinion appointment! Finally! But as this saga would have it, the appointment is scheduled for a day that I cannot be available. Andrew is trying to see if there is another November option that I could be there for, but I am doubtful—so here I am missing another appointment for work, but this conflict is not at my control and I am the only person who can tend to it. So I may miss it. My present question is, if this surgeon has Princess Pants as a patient, would they be planning for surgery now, or wait until she is in her teens? I am not even sure which answer I would prefer, but we will have seen our surgeon by then as well. So I may ask the same thing if I don't feel I am getting a straight answer. So there, good and bad, but progress none the less.

—Mom

ANDREW: WE'RE IN THE 21ST CENTURY, RIGHT?

October 17, 2014 (95 Days to Surgery)

It's not like we're just into the 21st century or anything. We're almost a full fourteen years into it and in trying to get Avery a second opinion with one of the most technologically advanced paediatric hospitals in the country what do we receive? A letter. Mailed to us with a stamp on it and everything.

In spite of the fact that I had left specific instructions with an actual human that I would like a phone call so that we can avoid any back and forth about times that work we get this letter. As Jodi mentioned, of course it's for one of the few times when she simply cannot make it. There wasn't many, but this was one of them.

So I call them back at the number provided in my mimeographed form letter and get voice mail. I left a message. The next day I call back again and have to leave another message. That afternoon I get a call back! It's someone asking about why I called and how they could help me. Strange, I was clear in my message I wanted to see if we could reschedule the appointment. "Oh! If you want to change your appointment you have to talk to [this other lady]! Let me transfer you." Voice mail. *sigh*

I leave a message. No response for the remainder of the day but lo and behold they called me back this morning! Turns out they can change the appointment but the doctor is only in once a week for this sort of thing and they're booked right up for a while. December 2nd is the earliest next appointment. Done. Good. Now let's move on, shall we?

Meeting with Avery's surgeon on Monday. Going to go over some things with her on the website he recommended and see if she has any questions. I know I have a big list of them piling up. I'm sure you'll see a few updates from us Monday afternoon / evening.

—Dad

THREE

MORE WAITING

A friend once told me that there's no point in worrying. The logic being that if you worry and everything works itself out in the end all you have done is make yourself suffer for no reason. Alternatively, if what you worry about comes true all you have done is suffer twice for the same thing. It is sound logic that I am incapable of putting into practice.

At this point it should be clear that the Canadian health care system, while great when it comes to costs, is less great when it comes to waiting. At practically zero, the price is right, but unless death is imminent you'd better grab a seat and have something to read. As someone with an overactive imagination and a strong sense of hypochondria this is a dangerous time. It gives the mind time to ponder what-ifs. It is where worrying takes a strange and unsettling form. I've been on Google; I know what's possible.

Here's a pro tip for parents and children alike: be careful what you Google. If you're not, it will send you down some rabbit holes that you don't want to go down.

I found that my biggest worry wasn't necessarily the one with the worst outcome. I've studied a bit of math in my time and I am aware of probabilities. Plus, I work for a health care company and risk assessment is a large part of what we do. The idea is that risks fit into a range that go from "broadly acceptable" to "patient will die," in Avery's case the likelihood of her dying on the table was minuscule, and even though the margin for error during the surgery is very small, the chance of her having mobility issues or becoming paralyzed were also small (one to four percent and one percent respectively).

My biggest worry was the one that was the most likely, especially when one considers Avery's specific case. Her spine angles were getting worse. I went looking at some doctor's websites that showed some before and after photos of various scoliosis patients and found some that were similar to Avery's. While the results were great there were quite a few that didn't get the spine perfectly straight again. In other cases, complications such as infection, pain due to the implants, or failure of the spine to fuse result in the need to undergo further surgeries. This was my biggest worry; that Avery would go through all this and still be left a little crooked or need to have surgery again.

It didn't matter to me that these cases were not Avery's. It didn't matter that these doctors were not Dr. Missiuna, or that the surgery didn't take place at Mc-Master Children's, or that every spine is unique and reacts differently to surgery, or that most data on complications are from older studies involving older surgical techniques. None of that mattered. The only thing my brain could think of was what would happen if they couldn't straighten her out? How would that impact her mental state? Her friendships? Her ability to function?

Sometimes more information doesn't feel like a good thing, and for a guy like me, the more waiting I did the more information I dug up. The more information I dug up the more worrying it was. It all started with the waiting, and there was still a whole lot of waiting to come.

This journey began in April 2014 and it was already October. That's six months of a whole lot of nothing going on for Jodi and I, and a birthday, an entire summer vacation, and the start of a new school year for Avery. So, how was Avery doing? This is more her story than anyone else's and you have only heard from her once up to this point.

How was she holding up?

Avery carried herself so well throughout this experience that it was often easy to forget that she was only eleven when this journey started. But, as good as Jodi and I were about keeping Avery informed every step of the way it would appear that she inherited some of her father's propensity for letting the what-ifs get to her. After the initial shock, it wasn't until mid-October that I started to see a crack in what seemed to be her impenetrable armor. That said, I also got a glimpse into her world of unbridled optimism.

AVERY: THE DAY BEFORE
October 19, 2014 (93 days to surgery)

I'm scared. I go for my third checkup tomorrow, where we'll hopefully find out when my surgery is, but I don't really want to because knowing when it's going to happen and knowing that it's going to happen are two very different things. But I'm afraid that if Dr. Missiuna doesn't tell us, my mom is going to rip off his head, because it's driving her crazy not knowing. Me? I'd be perfectly fine if no one ever told me when it was going to happen until I had to start donating blood, because if I haven't already said so I DON'T WANT TO KNOW!!!! Anyways, as I said at the beginning I don't want to know because knowing when just makes it all the more real. Talk to you more after the checkup.

—Princess Pants

JODI: PROGRESS
October 20, 2014 (92 Days to Surgery)

News! Results! And no, I wouldn't rip anyone's head off.

So first thing, my dad was a huge help spending the night so he could take the Dude to school, then he hung out here 'just in case the school called while we were away' which ended up being until nearly noon.

So on to McMaster. We arrived minutes before 8:00 (after getting lost. Perhaps we will use the GPS next time) to wait to get Pants' X-ray requisition—the receptionist let us in around 8:10 (I was totally pacing) and I budged in front of a brand new family there with their five-day-old baby. Jerk. I apologized—I was hoping to just grab the req and run over to X-ray, but we got fully checked in. Next time I will be more patient. On to X-ray, which was pretty uneventful and quick, then back to the clinic and we hardly sat down before we got called back (I think I prefer these 8:30 am appointments for that, though the inconvenience with Dude needs to be

45

balanced by my joy of not having to hang out in a hospital waiting room). We had a student doctor and a temperamental computer, so that stay was short, before we got sent back over for more X-rays in a bent over pose. We were back in the clinic and in front of the X-rays moments after returning to the clinic. There appeared to be progression of the curve, but the doctor didn't want to tell me us what the number was (but I saw it written down as ~60) which is roughly 18 degrees more than the first X-ray—without the 1 cm wood block correction since March.

This appointment I felt like I was getting more information—things like: surgery will be in January or February. She needs to have an MRI. Ok, maybe my head was going to pop off without more information. The doctor even suggested we visit his medical office, you know, just to show our faces—so we did. There we got a checklist with six things that need to happen before surgery. We told them that we would appreciate grouped appointments if possible so as to limit our travel. We were even offered paperwork for Ronald McDonald house, but I think we'll just do the drive and save that space for people who really need it.

And if that wasn't enough, by the time I was leaving the office tonight, we already had her MRI confirmed for this Sunday at 9:15 am—I mean wow! She doesn't even play professional sports.

So there. I feel like I know a little better what is coming and when it is coming. Avery seems okay, if not pleased, that she will make it through Christmas before surgery—and with this schedule, should be mostly healed up by the time summer vacation rolls around.

—*Mom*

AVERY: AFTER THE APPOINTMENT
October 21, 2014 (91 days to surgery)

So it's after the checkup and we found out the date. Well more information than we had. We found out that the surgery should happen around January/February so I will be able to have a normal Christmas. Yay! I can't wait till Halloween though, I'm going trick or treating with my friend! Oops, off track.

So anyways the doctor said that hopefully I'll be able to have my surgery in January/February, and that I have to have an MRI on Sunday. For the MRI I have to not move a muscle for forty minutes, and they figured that that would be hard for me so they're going to give me special goggles so that I can watch a movie. Yeah! But seriously, I'm not even going to be allowed to itch my nose! I bet that would be hard even for the most patient person! So more descriptive date, MRI on Sunday, check up in January, and that's all. You've been caught up. I'll talk more later. Bye.

—Princess Pants

JODI: MRI DONE
October 26, 2014 (86 Days to Surgery)

Avery had her MRI (I have said 'we had an MRI' a few times, but really, she was in alone) today. We were out the door by 8:15 for our 9:15 scheduled appointment in Hamilton. While in the Tim Hortons drive thru on our way there, I suddenly became concerned that maybe we needed to be there half an hour early for paperwork, but luckily my GPS had us set to arrive at 9:00, so I figured that split the difference.

We arrived around nine and parked in the blue section, right beside the elevator—such luck! Then we went to get the elevator to go up one level... and waited. Seriously, we waited maybe ten minutes. But there are no stairs in the blue level and never having been to blue, I was not sure on a Sunday at nine AM I could get from yellow to blue... so we waited. Finally in the elevator and up one floor to 1 where we needed to be buzzed in to the MRI section. On arrival, Tammy the MRI receptionist informed us that they had an emergency patient and were running fairly behind schedule, like at least two hours, and there was word that another emergency patient was coming down, so maybe three hours. We decided to wander the hospital, so now I know that McMaster is a box and you can in fact get all the way round, even on Sunday morning at 9:00 AM (and no paperwork needed. It seems the computers actually transmit information here).

After a half hour wander, we came back to see where things were at and were told we still had a couple of hours, but for certain 1 hour as both machines were in use, so we went to have breakfast at the Maple Leaf/Tally Ho Pancake house—the place where Andrew and I had breakfast the day we decided to date—19 years ago, almost exactly (October 20, 1994). I paid for our meal when I ordered in case we got a call to come back, so we just relaxed a bit—Avery was happy to eat peanut butter on her toast, a luxury she cannot have at home with her anaphylactic brother around. This pancake house is right beside Ronald McDonald House, and I am pretty sure the family that sat beside us was staying there. We headed back to the hospital, got the same parking spot! and a much quicker elevator ride back to the MRI area, Avery was given a lovely cotton hospital gown and before she could sit down, she was called back to her scan.

I made Avery wear yoga pants and a t-shirt and change her bra so she had no hooks because I recalled reading that she may have been able to wear her own clothes. Turns out I was misinformed because recent events have noted that many yoga pants contain silver threads—and they are not magnetic, but they are conductive and can apparently burn you. So no yoga pants. Cotton panties and a hospital gown to be safe. She also got to watch a movie while in there—how cool is that?

So 45 minutes, maybe an hour passed and out came a very flushed and very loopy Avery. She said she fell over and hit her head in the change room trying to put her sock on. After about five minutes I got up to check on her as she didn't have that much clothing to put back on. She was loopy. I had an MRI a couple of years ago, and I too was loopy, so at least I got it, but she was not pleased with the loopy feeling.

We left the hospital and went to a mall (her choice—she said she didn't want to go home yet) so I took her to Limeridge and we did a quick tour of the mall. I mentioned she was loopy? We went in to Gymboree (I really wanted the tie shirt for the Dude, but alas, none in his size) but while I was looking, she looked at the Eric Carle section, and they had the book Brown Bear, Brown Bear, What Do You See? And she lost it! She came over ranting about how it makes no sense! No sense at all! Then brought me over to explain—you see the first page reads "Brown Bear, Brown Bear what do you see? I see a red bird looking at me." the next page reads "Red Bird, Red Bird, what do you see" and here is where she lost it—the Red Bird sees a yellow duck! But the Brown Bear said the Red Bird was looking at him! So how can the Red Bird see something other than a Brown Bear?!? I really wish I had recorded it (but maybe that makes me a less than nice mother). This really bothered her, I mean even after we left the store, she continued to rant about it.

So really—the MRI was uneventful, as an MRI should be. I stopped by x-ray to see if I could pick up her x-rays for the Sick Kids appointment, but they were not there. So I asked to have the MRI put on a disk and we can take it too. And on the up side, the x-ray section was open, so theoretically, I can go pick the disks up on a Sunday morning between now and December 2.

—Mom

ANDREW: IT'S IN YOU TO GIVE

October 26, 2014 (86 Days to Surgery)

I want to talk about what happened last week and the profound impact it's had on me, and how I feel about charity and giving.

A few months ago a Facebook friend of ours had to have surgery. Brain surgery. Real dangerous stuff. He's the real estate agent who drove us around for two days back in 2009 and showed us almost thirty homes and ultimately helped us buy the house we have lived in for the past five years. He even did the final walk through so my wife and I wouldn't have to fly in from Ottawa to do it. We've stayed in touch on Facebook since then and followed the changes in his life, as he and his wife had their first child and then proudly announced earlier this year that another one was on the way.

During his surgery he almost died. He started to bleed and wouldn't stop. There was something like a 1% chance of this happening and it did. It took blood donations from sixty people to save his life. They pumped twelve litres of blood into him to keep him alive. Twelve litres. His body only holds four. He came out of surgery without a single drop of the blood he went in with—three times over.

Healing and grateful to be alive, he decided to give a little back and hold a blood drive down at the local Canadian Blood Services location in Waterloo and he asked all his friends on Facebook if they would consider donating.

I had low blood iron for the longest time and then was on some pretty fun medications after that and had never donated before. Being med free and with a healthy hemoglobin level right now the only thing stopping me was a healthy fear of needles and queasiness at the sight of blood, which seemed like really lame-ass excuses. So I booked my first ever appointment to donate blood for Tuesday of last week.

Then, in what can only be described as a karmic twist of the Universe, the Monday before my blood donation appointment Jodi and I found out that Avery does not weigh enough to bank her own blood before her surgery. It's a ten hour surgery and if not everything goes as planned she'll need blood. Better it's her own than someone else's too. Only now that was not possible.

Jodi cannot donate because of some funky rule that prohibits donations from people who lived in France for more than three months during certain years. Seeing as she lived there for a year during one of those years she's ineligible (something about mad cow disease and not being able to test for it until after you're dead). I will be tested for compatibility (blood type, antibodies, etc...) and if I'm a match I will provide a directed donation to have on hand for Avery's surgery. I'll only be able to donate a couple litres though. A worst case scenario would see her needing more than what I can offer.

That means there'll be blood on hand from the blood bank. I really hope none of it will be needed, but it's awfully reassuring that it's there if it is in fact needed.

So on Tuesday I went in and donated blood for the first time. It was almost completely painless, everyone was very supportive, and I got to have juice and cookies afterwards. My friend was even there talking with all the people donating and thanking them. If I'm being completely honest, I felt really good about it. The best way I can describe it was that I felt like I was making an immediate and profound impact on somebody's life. I went home afterwards proudly sporting my "First Time Donor" pin and feeling great (though getting out of bed the next morning was a challenge. I was really tired!)

I've been telling people this story ever since and am encouraging everyone to go find out if they are able to give blood, and if they are to please donate. It makes a difference. It saved my friend's life and could very well save Avery's.

—Dad

AVERY: GROWING UP SUCKS (SOMETIMES)
November 5, 2014 (76 Days to Surgery)

Growing up sucks. I wish we didn't have to grow up, because when you grow up everybody is always expecting you to try ten times as hard and never mess up. As you get older you have more responsibilities and a lot more people look up to you. A lot of the time I wish that I could have stayed eight forever, so that I wouldn't constantly have to be making sure I didn't mess anything up, because when you're older it seems that someone is always there waiting to criticize you every time you do even the smallest thing wrong. Teachers start telling you to forget stuff that's been nailed into your head since kindergarten, so that you can do it a way that's harder, you have to work out some things that other people have helped you with before on your own , and sometimes I just want to sit down and cry. Added to that, I have to worry about getting surgery. That's going to take a huge chunk out of my life, I mean, I'm not going to be able to do gym for a year, and I'm going to be off school for a month or more, so I'm going to miss a lot of things, and my internal organs will be all messed up because they will have more room to go where they're supposed to go. All in all I don't really want to grow up but if I don't grow up I'll never get to drive a car, or get a job, or go to high school or university , or become a teacher like I want to. If you don't grow up, you miss out on a lot of new things, but if you do, you're not supposed to do some things anymore, but you get to do new ones.

—Princess Pants

JODI: LATE NOVEMBER PROGRESS REPORT

November 26, 2014 (55 Days to Surgery)

Getting closer to having a date for surgery. The doctor's office advised they should have the January schedule by Friday- so we are either on it, or can be fairly confident it will be in February. But stuff is happening—Avery has her lung capacity test (required for surgery) on Monday morning and we go to Sick Kids on Tuesday.

I was hoping Avery would write about her upset at yoga last week, but I guess she is twelve—maybe her father can fill you in as he was there with her—what I got from the story was that Avery noticed her curve has gotten worse because they were doing some wall work, and previously she could do this stuff, but this time, she just couldn't. Since I like the silver lining for such things, I figure that a moment of personal recognition of the limitation at least makes all this talk of surgery not seem cosmetic or unnecessary in the eyes of the owner.

According to the Ontario wait time website, the average wait for this surgery at McMaster is 243 days. At Sick Kids it was over 400. Perspective helps I guess.

—Mom

FOUR

THE CLOCK STARTS

With Dr. Missiuna not doing surgery that month, Avery's would definitely happen sometime in the New Year. In fact, I found out after Avery's appointment that her condition had worsened to the point where she was at the top of the waiting list. The next time an operating room was allocated by the hospital for Dr. Missiuna to perform this surgery it would be Avery on the table.

This is when the rubber hits the road. Surgery would happen and happen soon. It was tangible. Real. Of course, it wasn't even remotely close to as real as it would get six weeks later, but at the time this was real life sweaty palms and yoga breathing anxiety management stuff. I'd like to say that the moments that were to come were the ones I'd trained for as a parent, but no one teaches you this stuff. I did manage to talk to a former colleague whose daughter had some spinal surgery and that was an educational experience I am glad I had the opportunity for.

"She'll be fine," was a statement he used quite a bit. "The doctors know what they're doing," was another. I was surprised at how relaxed he was when talking about his experiences. From my side of the table he looked cool as a cucumber and I was a pile of emotional jelly. It turned out that his daughter's surgery wasn't quite the same but it was pretty darn close and it was good to spend some time talking to someone who knew what I was going through. It was a great comfort.

After all the time that had passed there was one thing that bothered me. Avery still had not had a second opinion. Not that I didn't trust Dr. Missiuna. This wasn't his first rodeo, and his track record was perfect. But, it would be nice to have a second opinion. This was a big deal, and it was terrifying, and if there was even a remote chance to get another option I would have liked to hear it.

Looking back, I think the thing that was the hardest to process mentally was the fact that right out of the gate surgery was the only option. Believe me, I asked. Jodi asked. "But the internet says…!" I can't stress this enough: be careful what you Google. At the very least stay off Google if you're going out looking for that magic bullet that will make all of this go away. It doesn't exist. Yes, there are options out there that are not surgical. Yes, chiropractic care can provide some relief. Yes, yoga or physiotherapy can help and in some cases even reverse scoliosis.

Those were all things mentioned to me or to Jodi by people who weren't doctors. I appreciated their efforts, I really did. It was reassuring to know that when faced with no alternatives that they stepped up and tried to find some. They could see the panic in my eyes and the anxiety ripping through my body and they wanted to help, and they did help, but when you get down to it they weren't experts. I needed another person who has trained their entire adult life specifically for this purpose to look at my daughter and tell me what they would do if it was their child.

The score stood as follows: Surgery 1, Not Surgery 0. December would provide another tally and the fact that this book exists should tell you how that unfolded. In fact, December would be an eventful month, right down to finally getting a date for surgery and pre-op. Most importantly, Avery would get to have a normal Christmas.

ANDREW: OPINION SECONDED. MOTION CARRIED

December 2, 2014 (49 Days to Surgery)

Driving to Toronto sucks.

Today was the day that months of waiting finally paid off as we travelled to our much anticipated second opinion appointment with a surgeon at the Hospital for Sick Children ("Sick Kids") in Toronto.

As it turned out, months and months of waiting culminated with hours and hours of waiting. Our appointment was for 10:00 and we were told to be there at 9:30. We got Jodi's dad to come over last night so we could leave early enough in the morning and he could take The Dude to school for 8:30. We left a smidge after 7:30 and got to Sick Kids at 9:38.

Did I mention that driving to Toronto sucks?

We arrive at the orthopaedic clinic at 9:40 and wait in line until 10:00. After a good fifteen minutes to get registered and get all of the images copied over from CD we go off to x-ray, where we wait some more. From x-ray we go back to orthopaedics and we wait there, and wait, and wait, and wait. Sometime around 11:50 we get to go to a room! We wait there for another ten minutes or so before we are greeted by a very pleasant Nurse Practitioner named Kim (I believe it was Kim. Jodi noticed her name but I only got her title. All you psychology/sociology nerds can judge me later, I'm telling a story here).

Nurse Practitioner Kim was wonderful with Avery and put her through a barrage of tests, the whole time telling us that she had spoken with the surgeon and would be bringing him in shortly. At around 12:25 or so Kim left to get the surgeon and I ran out to put more money in the S.S. Minnow parking meter thingy (it only lets you pay in three hour tours).

The surgeon returned a few minutes after I got back and gave us the news that we knew was coming: the only way to fix Avery's curve is through surgery. This was not unexpected but I know that I found it reassuring nonetheless.

We did find out a few other things while we were there as well:

• Her spine is probably only going to grow another couple centimetres so this is a good time to have the surgery (she's going to be all legs, just like her mother).

• Spine angles in her range typically get 70-80% corrected (as opposed to only 50% correction if her angles were worse).

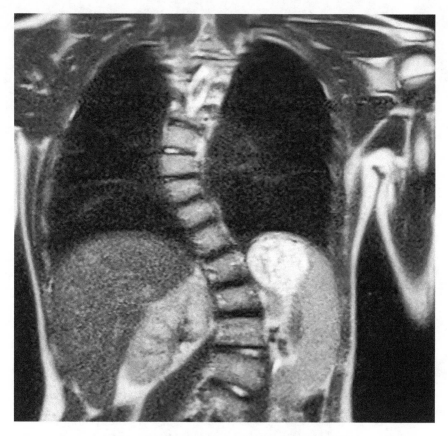

MRI image, October 26, 2014. (Personal Medical Record)

• *The doctor feels she has more flexibility than she was showing during her bend tests today (anxiety and having been sitting in a car and chairs all morning factors).*

• *She's not likely going to need a brace after her surgery (they only brace afterwards in a select few cases).*

• *Her spine is also rotated (in addition to curved). Rotation of the spine for a curve this large is expected and they'd be worried if it didn't.*

And that was that. Since this was a second opinion appointment there wasn't any further paperwork required and she was discharged and off we went. To give you some of an idea of what Avery's spine looks like now I took this low-res screen shot off my laptop from her MRI on October 26:

As you can see, there's no doubt about it. Because of the "S" curve in her spine she bends to one side better than she does the other. As Jodi alluded to in a previous post Avery and I were at yoga two weeks ago and Avery tried to do some wall work (yoga against a wall—it's much harder and gives you an indication of your true range of motion). Well, she was unable to do a posture that she previously had no trouble with. It was the first physical manifestation of her condition that she had experienced and it was in front of a whole bunch of people she didn't know. This brought on a wave of emotions and she broke down in the middle of class and I had to bring her home. As a parent it was incredibly hard for me to watch so I can only imagine how hard it was for her to experience. Anyway, she went back next week with my mother and they didn't do wall work and they both had a great time.

Up next: On Thursday Avery does her cardio-pulmonary baseline tests and afterwards she gets her blood and antibodies typed and I get my blood tested for compatibility.

—Dad

JODI: A DATE! (MAYBE)

December 11, 2014 (40 Days to Surgery)

We might have a date! January 26, 2015 if the hospital confirms. Seven weeks. This could all be happening in seven weeks. And Andrew can direct donate as his blood and antibodies are a match—I can't because of the mad cow disease thing. So once we know if we are confirmed—hopefully by Monday, then things just start happening. Including a trip to Great Wolf Lodge for just before, because why not.

Seven weeks!

—Mom

JODI: WE HAVE A DATE!

December 17, 2014 (34 Days to Surgery)

After a torturous week of back and forth with the surgeon's office and the hospital and Andrew (probably better for everyone this has been with Andrew and not me) we have a confirmed date for the surgery. January 20th. Like a month from now. I am very happy that the first big wait is done and we can now start some concrete planning, but now we have the big wait for the day to actually arrive. Between now and then we have an appointment with the surgeon to discuss the MRI and some surgery details, a meeting with the hospital appointed social worker, Andrew will donate three units of blood for use if necessary for Avery in the surgery, a pre-op day, and I promised an overnight to Great Wolf Lodge. I suppose I should also plan on a trip to the school to ensure things are in place for her school work while she is recovering. The next 33 days are going to be busy. As are the next four months while she is recovering.

All the positive thoughts in the world are welcome, in whatever format works for you that this all goes as planned and Avery is walking around the house before February arrives.

—Mom

AVERY: AAAAAHHHHHHHHHHHH!

December 17, 2014 (34 Days to Surgery)

I just got back from yoga and found out that the surgery will happen on the twentieth of January. Six days earlier than we thought. I don't really know what I'm feeling, because I don't want to scream or cry. I cried a little at the start, but now I'm not sure. I guess I just want to process it, get it through my head that a bunch of people I don't know are going to CUT A HOLE IN MY BACK WHILE I'M ASLEEP. Ok well now I want to scream, but at least we have a date. A definite date. No backing out now. I'm going to get surgery. "Yah!"

—Princess Pants

JODI: PRE-OP CONFIRMED. I GUESS WE'RE DOING THIS

December 23, 2014 (28 Days to Surgery)

Pre-op is scheduled for January 13. Great Wolf Lodge is booked for January 15/16 and we are bringing two of Avery's friends (I am sure they are upset about the day off school to go to a waterpark). So it seems like everything is rolling out as it should, and once the holidays are over, the surgery will come quick (maybe faster than we are emotionally ready for, but there is nothing to be done about that).

We will work out the details with my parents for the week Avery will be in the hospital so that the Dude is well cared for and not left standing on the curb at school waiting for me to show up.

Four weeks today.

—Mom

Andrew: The Countdown Is On... And Dad Chimes In Again

December 29, 2014 (22 Days to Surgery)

Well it's been a pretty hectic last couple weeks. I wanted Jodi (who was growing frustrated with each passing minute with no date) and Avery (who is understandably terrified and going through this on a level that I can't even begin to understand) to get their thoughts out while I took it all in and processed it.

I've been meaning to post and then kept putting it off not thinking I had anything worthwhile to say. It's a lot of worrying. Nothing I can do but reassure Avery that she's in great hands and that she's a strong girl who will handle this like a champ. Still, it's on my mind pretty much all the time. I distract myself with work and anything I can, but the second I let my guard down it's on my mind—and it's crushing me.

The biggest part is I can't do anything. It's hard to describe, this feeling of being the father. I didn't get to carry her in my womb for eight-and-a-quarter months. I don't know what it's like to have that connection that mothers have with their children. The list of things I am clueless about is extensive.

I can be there for her, emotionally and to hold her hand or give her a hug, and that's what I plan on doing as much as I possibly can. I can also donate blood, though for much of today it looked like that wasn't going to happen. I got a voice mail today from Canadian Blood Services saying that due to a scheduling problem they wouldn't be able to get me in to provide a donation.

I'll be completely honest. I was really upset. This was to be the one thing that I could actually do for Avery and I was really looking forward to doing it. Knowing that if something happened during surgery and they needed blood that mine would be the first drops they would go to, well, it was an indescribable feeling, and with one voice mail that rug was pulled out from under me. Not quite devastating, but pretty darn close. The message said I should call them back, so I did, but I got voice mail. A few minutes later I got a call back from a coordinator saying that her manager would be calling me back to explain.

While doing the dishes that night I got a call from Canadian Blood Services. The manager informed me that they would be able to fit my donation into the schedule: January 8th, with details to follow. What makes me feel really good about this is that the gentleman who called said that the problem with scheduling came to his attention at 1:00 and he's been working on rejigging the schedules because, "We really wanted to make sure you were able to make this donation for your daughter."

Faith in the system restored.

So, it seems like getting to a surgery date is the biggest hurdle because once you have a date, boy howdy do things ever move like clockwork. Surgical consult within three weeks of getting the date; blood donation two days after that; pre-op booked for a week before the surgery, and several weeks in advance...

It's very encouraging, if not a bit overwhelming.

So there you have it, a ridiculously busy January on the horizon.

—Dad

FIVE

THE FINAL COUNTDOWN

After a whirlwind December, January brought a solid dose of reality. It was no longer necessary to use all my fingers and toes to count down the days and Avery was understandably terrified. It is from here that Avery would go exactly one month between blog posts (for obvious reasons, as you will soon read) whereas Jodi and I would crank out thirty-three posts between us.

As a parent, seeing one of my children in pain and afraid is the hardest thing I have ever had to deal with. In the few weeks leading up to the surgery I was an absolute mess. As someone with a history of hypochondria, anxiety, and insomnia, I was uncertain how I would hold up. It turns out that the answer to that was, 'not well', but at the same time I can honestly say that the answer was also, 'better than I thought I would'.

For the first nineteen days of the year, the ones leading up to the surgery date, I managed only one post. If I'm being completely honest, I wasn't my sharpest at the office either. The issues I had to deal with at the office were minuscule compared to what my daughter was about to go through. Heck, the issues of THE WORLD seemed small at the time.

If I'm the anxious worrier of the family then Jodi's the pragmatic emotional rock. We're a good match in that at any moment we'll have the entire spectrum of emotions covered. Ever see one of those cheesy movies or TV shows where someone is running around all panicked and someone else grabs them by the shoulders, stops them from moving, and then slaps them in the face while yelling, "Snap out of it!"? Well, I was the one spinning around in circles and Jodi was the one slapping me in the face. I have found that it is good to have someone like this close to me and it is part of the reason Jodi and I have been together for more than two decades.

It was important for me that we didn't hide our emotions. Yes, Jodi did a wonderful job of tempering and adding perspective, but as a family we made sure not to suppress what we were feeling. It's the reason I think the blog was such a success for us. It allowed everyone to release what they were thinking and feeling out into the world. It was a cathartic exercise of letting go and moving on.

It was also a time that highlighted all the wonderful people there are in the world, in particular those close to us. If I were giving advice to families going through a similar experience it would be to open yourselves up to people however you can. What you get back in compassion from others will fill your soul with confidence and fill your heart with strength.

Not mentioned in the one blog post I did leading up to the surgery was the fact that I was able to do my blood donation. Along with the tiara incident which you'll read about shortly, my blood donation was another happy highlight.

I drove the hour from my house down to the blood bank near the hospital and waited my turn. I did the requisite finger prick check on my hemoglobin and found that it was a bit low. Not so low that they wouldn't let me donate, but at the absolute minimum required. I was asked if I was sick. I had a bit of a cold coming on, I thought, said that overall was feeling pretty good. Which I was, but hoped they would still let me donate.

They did.

The weird thing about doing the directed donation—one that goes from a specific person to another specific person as opposed to in the general bank— was that they had to do a lot of paperwork. In hindsight it made a lot of sense because every rule they had to keep donors and recipients anonymous had to be "broken" in order to guarantee that the blood they took from me ended up in Avery and no one else. And there were a lot of precautions taken to ensure that it went exactly as planned. I was given a ticket, something that looked like I had just bought into the 50/50 draw at my local community centre.

This ticket was the most important part of the whole process. I gave it to the admitting nurse at the hospital the morning of the surgery. It was what matched up my blood with Avery's operating room. I put the ticket in my wallet and then put my wallet in my front pocket. I would not let that wallet out of my sight for the next seven days.

I'd like to take this moment to thank all the people at Canadian Blood Services, specifically all the ones at their Hamilton location. They do absolutely wonderful work and along with the donors they are the reason that so many people are alive today. The manager who rejigged the schedule so I could give blood to Avery even showed up for my donation so he could make sure I was being taken care of. With my mind in a hundred places I didn't get his name and I feel terrible about that, but the fact that he did all he could for me and then showed up to personally see it through is testament to the amount he cared and the level of care you receive from everyone at Canadian Blood Services.

I'd like to also take a moment to thank all of Avery's teachers and classmates who were at Hespeler Public School for the 2013/2014 school year. Those kids showed more compassion than I have ever seen and it still brings a tear to my eye when I think about it. Five days a week Jodi and I had to send Avery off to school and we had to go to work. That made it very hard to keep an eye on Avery to see how she was doing. Knowing that all of her classmates and teachers had her back during the day was a big relief. You'll read about a few times in the next couple months where these kids stepped up and made a big difference, not just for Avery but for Jodi and myself as well.

AVERY: I'M SCARED

January 3, 2015 (17 Days to Surgery)

I'm scared that it hurts when I stand for too long. That it hurts when I put on my socks or tie my shoes without sitting. I'm terrified that one day I'm just going to wake up and find out that the surgery happened and now I have to heal it all. I'm terrified to cry. Because whenever I feel like crying, I also feel like everyone is going to laugh. And then when I finish crying, I feel really stupid. I know that after my family reads this they're going to be like, "Oh, Avery you have a right to be sad. Go ahead and cry, no one will laugh". And I know that that's probably true but it doesn't make it any less scary. It just makes me think that there's all the more reason to be scared.

    Anyways, that's all.

—*Princess Pants*

AVERY: STATISTICS

January 5, 2015 (15 Days to Surgery)

    2.0% of girls between the ages of eight and eighteen are affected by scoliosis. 0.5% of boys between those ages are affected by scoliosis. Together that means that 2.5% of children between eight and eighteen years of age are affected by scoliosis. That's only three out of every two hundred people and about 17,500,000 out of the whole world. In percentages it seems really small, but when you look at the grand scheme of things, you realize that lots of people have it. Some people may only have very minor curves while others look really funky. I know I'm not the only one, but sometimes it feels like it. I have surgery in 16 days but it still feels like a bad dream that I'm just about to wake up from. It just started feeling real last night, but I'm still hoping that I'll just wake up.

    I wish I could.

—*Princess Pants*

JODI: T MINUS 14

January 6, 2015 (14 Days to Surgery)

    We saw the surgeon today—the last time before surgery. Avery got in some bonus round x-rays and measured in at 62°. Today's x-rays took forever—or about an hour, but I am certain we have never waited longer than twenty minutes—I mean we took so long, the surgeon came in to x-ray to find us.

    We had time for a few questions, and then the surgeon stopped us to ask about Avery's injections, to which we all looked at him a little puzzled. Turns out ideally she would have started these Eprex injections a couple of weeks ago to help stimulate her red blood cell and bone marrow growth in advance of her surgery. So we left with a prescription and instruction to start this today with her family doctor, and if that wasn't possible, to head back to Hamilton tomorrow so he could do it.

I should have realized that this was not going to be easy by that offer. I was driving, so I had Andrew call the nurse to ask if this could be done. When she called back, it was a little special, and is normally administered in a hospital, so she needed to get clearance to do it. After we got home, she called back and said they could do it at 2:50 PM today. This was at about 2:00 PM.

Next up, I thought perhaps I should call and confirm if the pharmacy had some. I called ours—no go. I called the Shopper's down the road—no go. I called the other pharmacy down the road—no go, but that pharmacist at least had a suggestion, so I followed it. Success at the Preston Medical Pharmacy! Though there was no way we were going to make it to the doctor's office for 2:50 PM.

In the end, we made it by 3:45 PM, including a stop for cat food and to our normal pharmacy to transfer the scrip over so the next week's dose isn't such an adventure. She was called in almost immediately, and as fate would have it, the nurse who was administering the drug had spinal fusion surgery just last year. She said she'd be the one giving her the needle next week too, so if Avery thinks of any questions, she should just bring them with her.

And as the day ended, my MIL came by to bring Avery a prayer shawl. T minus 13.

—Mom

JODI: T MINUS 7

January 13, 2015 (7 Days to Surgery)

We had Avery's pre-op appointment today—after a slight detour home when Andrew asked if I had the pre-op yellow envelope and I realized it was at home still.

Anyway, we were only minutes late with that detour and were in to see the first person—the Child Life Specialist. She was lovely and walked Avery through the day of surgery. She also warned Avery that hospitals can be quite boring so she should pack lots of entertainment—feel free to comment with any ideas to help her pass her days—thanks to a hefty Christmas haul she just bought seven new books, but she has lots of iTunes money to download or rent movies with, as well.

Next up was her first health study invitation—this one is apparently worth four hours towards the forty volunteer hours required to graduate high school, but I am not sure if she can accumulate high school volunteer hours while still in grade seven. This study is aiming to better understand immune-metabolic connections to health and study of the role of the immune system on body weight and metabolism.

Then we saw the nurse. She was lovely and went over her bits, then ended to take some blood from Avery.

While the blood work was happening, we were approached for a second survey focusing on pain management during scoliosis surgery and treatment. This one comes with a $10 gift card for one of three places. After a failed first attempt at blood collection, the nurses had success and we were back in the waiting area.

A few minutes later we were into see the anesthesiologist. We expressed the potential allergy to anectine, but we're assured that it would not be used for this surgery and in fact is rarely used at all these days.

And then we were done. We are due back at 6:30 am on Tuesday, January 20th for surgery. One of us can sleep at the hospital with her all week. We'll see what makes sense for us.

Now it is just enjoying this week. Great Wolf Lodge is in 48 hours so I think we will focus on that.

I am hoping Avery will let me take some before photos—so we can tell the full story once this is over. She did measure in at 5' 4" today—and will likely be 5' 6" this time next week.

(She did let me take some photos)

—Mom

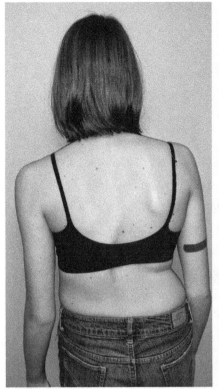 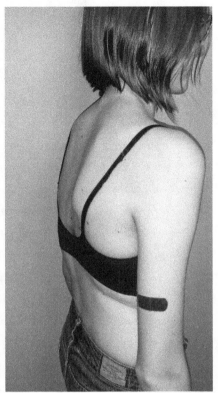

Seven Days Before Surgery. (Family Photos)

ANDREW: OVERWHELMING SHOW OF SUPPORT

January 17, 2015 (Three Days to Surgery)

So we're down to just a few days before surgery and on Thursday Pants had her last day of school. Before we get to the awesomeness that was Thursday let me first say that the support that we have received from friends, family, colleagues, and their friends, family and colleagues has been overwhelming. However people have chosen to put wellness, love, and positive thoughts into the world, they have done it in spectacular fashion. There have been prayers, cards with wonderful thoughts, iTunes and Chapters gift cards, a pat on the back, a genuine smile, hands to hold, and lots of hugs. Overwhelming. Oh, and there were tiaras.

Tiaras? Yep, because our daughter whom we affectionately call Pants isn't just Pants. Her official nick name is Princess Pants. Her name actually started out as Princess Paloney Baloney but has since evolved. The point being she's our little princess and princesses wear tiaras (duh!)

We decided as a family to pull Pants and a couple of her friends out of school on Friday so we could take them to Great Wolf Lodge indoor water park for a bit of fun. The surgery is on Tuesday and we weren't about to make her go to school on the Monday so that made Thursday her last day of school before the surgery.

For her last day of school before surgery Princess Pants decided that she was going to wear a tiara—just because she could. Her two Great Wolf Lodge friends, in a show of support, also decided that this should be a thing and agreed to wear one as well. Before too long the teacher found out, and then the rest of her class and what they did brought a tear to my eye.

The whole lot of them, even the boys, donned tiaras for a class photo!

Unfortunately I don't think I can post the photo here as we didn't get permission from all the other kids' parents to put their picture on the internet but I can tell you that it's truly a beautiful sight.

Thanks to those who provided some headgear, thanks to her class for being such a great bunch of kids, thanks to the teachers for going along with it, thanks to her friends for being such great friends, and thanks to everyone for being so supportive.

—Dad

JODI: ADVENTURES IN PHARMACEUTICALS
January 18, 2015 (2 Days to Surgery)

Tomorrow is supposed to be Avery's third and final Eprex injection. Supposed to be. Andrew ended up getting the groceries yesterday—I don't even know why, but as a result of it not being me, nothing triggered a stop at the pharmacy. A few hours later, I asked him, and of course he did not stop—and I thought at that moment that I should call them to make sure all was good as we had some challenges last week—but it slipped my mind. I had planned to pick it up today, so after some adventures in hair dye, Avery and I went out at 4:30—noting the pharmacy closes at 5:00 so it needed to be our first stop.

We went to the pick-up counter, and asked for her script, pointing out it is refrigerated. Nothing. Not even a non-prescribed one like last week. So I speak with the pharmacist. I explained that when I picked it up last Sunday, I ordered the refill for today. I spoke with both the pharmacist and the tech. The tech even took part of the scrip print-out 'to make sure the details are correct.'

The pharmacist (who has been our pharmacist since 2000) was very upset. He called every pharmacy in the city, but as my experience showed two weeks ago, no one had this drug in the required dose. He then called his pharmacy rep and pleaded with her to get someone over to the warehouse. In the end he asked for my cell number and promised to text me once he had confirmation.

I got the text at 5:47 stating that the courier will be delivering the needle around 8 (and the pharmacist will be in an hour early to get it) and he will text me once he has it in his hands tomorrow. He apologized again and thanked me for my patience.

So it will all work out. Just like this whole surgery thing will.

—Mom

SIX

A DIFFERENT KIND OF WAITING

The surgery was scheduled for first thing in the morning. This meant that we had to be at the hospital for 6:30 AM., which is an early start for everybody especially when you consider we all needed to drag our butts out of bed and then drive forty-five minutes down to the hospital. I did not sleep the night before. I tried, but woke up too frequently for any of the sleep I did get to matter. Jodi was the same way. Avery claims to have slept but I'm not sure I believe her.

Jodi's dad came over to stay with our son, AJ, and we were out the door well before six o'clock. I don't even remember if AJ was awake when we left or not. We wanted to make sure that everything was as normal as possible for him so staying at home and sleeping in his own bed and keeping his own routine was of paramount importance. This turned out to be a wonderful idea and it allowed us to free up a room at Ronald McDonald house for a family that was in greater need.

So, the big day was upon us and I was in the passenger seat. Avery was in back listening to her Vance Joy and Taylor Swift music and Jodi was driving. It was quiet but you could hear lots of deep breaths coming from everyone every couple minutes. I'm happy the hospital was as close to our house as it was because I'm not sure I could have made it through any more driving without turning into a puddle on the floor mat. Still it was forty-five minutes of staring out the window and waiting.

We were told that one parent would get to go into the surgical theatre with Avery. Jodi said she couldn't do it so it was I who got to make the long walk with her into the operating room. Everything had to be ready and I had to wear this wonderful getup to keep all my hair and germs and stuff out of the room. Of course, I had to wait. Yay, more waiting! This time I got to wear some sort of biohazard suit that wasn't designed to be worn for very long. It wasn't exactly the most breathable outfit I've ever had on.

From the date of first diagnosis to the day of the surgery was 295 days with most of that spent waiting. You would think that at this point I would be getting good at it. Well, surgery waiting was MUCH different than any other waiting. Jodi and I had to pack enough supplies to keep us comfortable and occupied for at least ten hours, and then we had to sit and wait, or pace and wait, or wander aimlessly though the cold, sterile halls and wait.

Adding to the stress of the day was the fact that my parents were in Barbados and my brother's wife was due to give birth at any moment. I figured my mom must have been a basket case so we had a video call scheduled for 9:00 PM to go over the day's events.

Technology for the win!

I have always been a bit of a social media nerd, particularly Twitter and Facebook, but it wasn't until the surgery day that I discovered its true usefulness. In addition to having a video call with my mother from inside the Paediatric ICU, I managed four blog posts on the day with a fifth coming after twenty-four hours at the hospital. There was an outpouring of support on Facebook from friends both old and new, and Twitter provided an endless stream of material to keep me distracted.

That said, I spent most of the day in the same chair watching people in the waiting room come and go. I stopped counting after a while, but I can say that gallbladder surgeries are quite popular and don't take very long at all. Tonsils are another big one. There were lots of tonsils being removed that day. And then there was Jodi and I, in for the long haul. If I had to do it again I would bring a pillow and make sure I had a warm, hooded sweatshirt with me. Of course, I packed a bunch of things to have on hand but I forgot those two items, both of which would have proved invaluable.

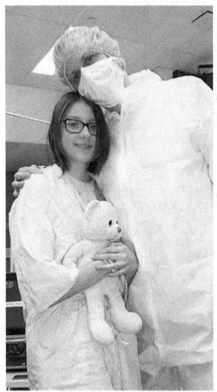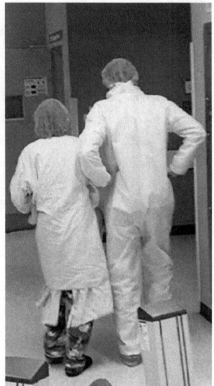

Avery and Andrew in the pre-op waiing room and walking back to the surgical suite. (Family Photo)

My advice for anyone sitting in the waiting room while their child is in for a long-haul surgery is plain and simple: *Keep yourself distracted.*

Sitting there staring at the clock on the wall is not going to make the surgery go any faster, nor will it have some magical effect on the surgeons working. Everyone working on fixing your child is a trained professional and many of them have been doing this for a long time. Do whatever activity works best for you to pass the time.

That said, no matter what you do it is going to feel like time is barely moving.

It's okay.

Really.

Breathe.

Your child is in good hands.

ANDREW: T MINUS 2H 9MIN

January 20, 2015 (2 Hours to Surgery)

In the car on the way to the hospital. Avery slept well but admitted to waking at 11:30 to get her last sip of water for a while and to have a good cry.

Jodi says she did not sleep very well. I know because I saw every hour on the clock and she was tossing and turning quite a bit.

Our ETA is about half an hour and we should arrive before our scheduled 6:30 AM appointment. I will be taking her in to be sedated at 8:00 AM and then the longest ten hours I can imagine begins.

More later. Thanks for thinking of us.

—Dad

ANDREW: AND SO IT BEGINS

January 20, 2015 (2 Hours Into Surgery)

One parent gets to come into the operating room with the child. Guess who it was?

As you can see they give you some fancy clothes and a cool hair net (shoe booties not shown). The anesthesiologist came to say hello and explain everything. Then the surgeon, Dr. Missiuna, came to say hello and ask how Pants was doing. Then a nurse came by and we were off to the OR. Avery is going to be in one of the new ones so I was expecting a lot of fanciness. I was not disappointed.

The OR was filled with all kinds of machines and tables and people. Lots and lots of people. At one point I counted ten!

The nurses got her all hooked up with an oxygen meter on her finger, some sticky pads on her chest and back for some machine (hopefully the one that goes "ping!"), and then the anesthesiologist started her IV. She was worried about the needle but they numbed her up pretty good. He gave her some calming medicine and she started to cry. We just practiced our breathing, eyes fixed on each other, me trying to make mine smile so she could see that everything would be okay. Then the first dose of sleepy time medicine was pushed through and she was out a few seconds later. They let me give her *a kiss and then a nurse walked me back to Jodi. All in all I think I was in there for ten minutes but let me tell you that it was the longest and most emotional ten minutes of my entire life.*

Now we wait.

They gave us a pager in the event we're not in the family waiting room and the doctor wants to talk to us. We can also request updates and have them relayed back to us from the OR.

How long do we have to wait before the surgery is done?

TEN hours.

The longest ten freaking hours of our lives.

Two shifts of volunteers are going to come and go and we'll still be here, waiting.

—

At 9:20, about an hour after I left the OR, Dr. Missiuna came into the waiting room. He said rather quickly that it was just an update so we'd know what was going on but it wasn't quick enough to prevent the heart attack upon seeing him.

He was just letting us know that Bruno the anesthesiologist was done and now it was his turn. I guess prep takes about an hour—which Dr. Missiuna said it would—as they have to get her a central line (in her neck), another IV, a catheter, a breathing tube, and then plug her into all the machines.

Now we wait.

—

Random notes:

• Jodi picked up a parking pass so we don't have to spend $20/day for the week we're here.

• One of the researchers came by to pick up the paperwork Pants and Jodi filled out.

• I ate a bagel and had some juice but still feel sick to my stomach.

• I almost cry when I read all the wonderful comments on Facebook, Twitter, and text messages.

• I am really happy that "anesthesiologist" is one of the first words autocorrect suggests.

— Dad

ANDREW: MORE THAN HALFWAY?

January 20, 2015 (6.5 Hours Into Surgery)

If all goes as planned we're more than halfway through.

Here are some random thoughts:

• I've lost count of the number of people who've already come and gone from the waiting room.

• There's a big clock on the wall that I glance at every now and then too. By "now and then" I mean at least once every 2.5 seconds.

• We're not asking the OR for updates. Instead we're taking the no news is good news approach. Business as usual for the experts.

• I managed to eat some lunch and read lots of comments on Facebook.

• Just noticed that my hands are freezing but my pits are sweaty.

• I ate peanut M&M's (because The Dude is at home and I'll be here all day and night) and they were absolutely fantastic!

• Our friend Pete changed his profile pic to him wearing a tiara. Pete is awesome.

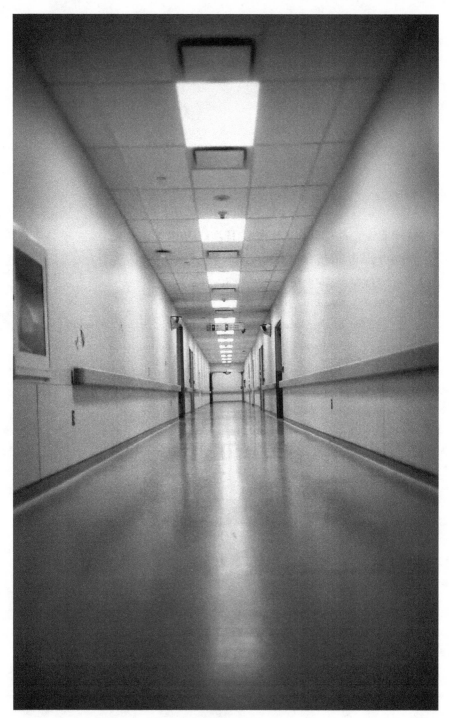

The long, empty hallway. (Andrew Butters)

• Our friend Jay called while away on business just because he figured I'd need a distraction (he was right).

• There is this really long empty hallway around the corner. It's a little creepy.

That's it for now. Another update to come when there's an update to give.

—Dad

JODI: PASSING THE TIME. LOTS OF TIME.
January 20, 2015 (8 Hours Into Surgery)

We are on to the second shift of hospital volunteer in the OR waiting room. And down to 3 people waiting, though two of them are the other parent/person waiting. I asked the hospital volunteer when her shift was over, as the morning lady told us it would be before Avery is out of surgery—she kindly offered to stay after her shift so we could eat a little later (this almost made me cry) as she lives both close and alone, so she really didn't mind. Oh, the dilemma.

I tried to update Avery's classmates—though I am not sure that a few of them still don't think it was Avery just speaking about herself in the third person.

Time passes very slowly here. But my step count is over 5k. :)

—Mom

ANDREW: THE FINAL COUNTDOWN
January 20, 2015 (9 Hours Into Surgery)

Here we are.

Eleven hours at the hospital and Avery has been in surgery for almost nine. I'll be honest, I'm a bit anxious and I'm exhausted. Completely exhausted. We still haven't heard word from the OR and we're taking that as a really good sign. Every time someone walks by the windows though I look up and hope it's Dr. Missiuna.

There's a hospital worker doing laps wearing her headphones. I think she's on lap nine or ten.

Dawn was the lovely old lady on shift two for the volunteers. She was supposed to leave at 4:30 but stuck around to see another woman to her kid and another man in to wait (we have company now!) and she absolutely insisted we go eat. Wouldn't leave until we did. So we ate and she left (but not before asking if I wanted another warm blanket—such a sweet woman). The new guy in the waiting room is playing a game on his iPhone that dings every ten seconds. I am annoyed but too polite to say anything.

Hot in Cleveland *is on the TV.*

Next update likely won't be until Avery is set up in the ICU. Breathing in. Breathing out.

—Dad

SEVEN

EVERYTHING IS OKAY, BUT...

Want to know the worst word in the English language? *But.* And there it was, hanging off the nurse's tongue like a poison pill. "The surgery went well, *but....*" and that's when my eyes widened. If time was barely moving while I was sitting in the waiting room then it came to a complete stop as soon as I heard the word *but.* I had not prepared for a *but.* I had also not prepared myself for what Avery was going to look like in the hours immediately after the surgery.

It was explained to us by Dr. Missiuna that Avery would be swollen from the anaesthetic. It was also explained to us that the surgery was most comparable to getting hit by a truck. It was one of the most invasive surgeries that you could perform on a person. Other people had told me that she would look swollen or "different" after the surgery as well, but I never really asked anyone what that meant.

So, when the Pediatric ICU nurse came in to talk to us and explained that she was covered in hives from her knees to her neck it was a punch that hit me right in the gut and took the air out of my lungs. As someone with a son with an anaphylactic allergy (peanuts) as well as one himself (shellfish) I know how serious this is.

The good news was since Avery was already intubated, she was breathing fine and her oxygen levels were still good. The bad news was they had no idea what caused the reaction and they were going to keep her sedated and intubated for another twelve hours.

Oh, and she looks like she's been hit by a truck.

It had been more than twelve hours since we last saw Avery. It was twelve hours of pure anxiety and when I walked into her ICU room that anxiety turned to shock. Looking back, I can see why television shows dramatize reunions with loved ones coming out of surgery. "That's not my husband!" the person screams as they run over and grab the hand of the poor soul lying in bed all bruised, battered, and bandaged.

The hit-by-truck analogy was accurate. The skin had worn off parts of her face from all the jostling and rubbing against the operating room table. There were three IVs doing various things and she was hooked up to several machines. Avery was intubated, which was the first time I had ever seen someone in that state before. It was unsettling, to say the least.

Dripping from the catheter was nuclear green pee. Hives covered Avery's chest and arms and I'm told they extended all the way down to her knees, which also sported scrapes from lying face down on the table for ten hours. Those scrapes were apparently part of a matching set of six to go along with the two on her face and two more on Avery's hips.

My daughter was unconscious and it looked like she was being kept alive by machines. Jodi and I were assured that Avery was doing just fine on her own and that the machines were just monitoring her progress and medication levels. With the exception of the hives, everything was normal.

It would be twelve hours before they would wake Avery up and remove her breathing tube.

JODI: THROUGH THE WOODS, BUT NOT QUITE OUT OF THEM

January 20, 2015 (11 Hours of Surgery + 1 Hour Post Op)

Surgery lasted an hour and eighteen minutes longer than planned. That was a stupid long extra 78 minutes to this already seriously long day. And then it gets worse. We still haven't seen her. Her surgeon has been by and said all the reassuring things the surgeon is supposed to say, and the receiving Pediatric ICU nurse did a debrief. The debrief included letting us know Pants is allergic to something she came in contact with today, so she is covered in hives, but as she is still intubated, her breathing is fine. She also advised that her pee is green from the drugs that are keeping her unconscious. She will be kept out for 24 hours—that too seems like more than I was planning on, but if that is what she needs, I am all for it. She also told us her eyes are swollen shut from being facedown all day, that we were told about—I'll let you know how it really is when we see her.

So now we wait. Anxiously. Another waiting room, another wait.

—Mom

JODI: 4:32 AM FROM THE PEDIATRIC ICU
January 21, 2015 (+6 Hours Post OP)

Avery needed this surgery. It wasn't cosmetic. If it wasn't done she would have possibly had difficulty breathing and it would have impacted her for her whole life. I have to tell you, though, seeing her in the Pediatric ICU hooked up to monitors and a ventilator and looking like she has just lost a boxing match is making me feel sick. She is heavily sedated and her wrists are tied down to the bed so she doesn't pull the intubation tube out. I am up now because there was just a flurry of activity because she is running a fever, so the nurse wanted to give her some Tylenol and flip her over to her left side.

To survive the surgery, Avery not only needed the blood donation Andrew provided, but three or four times what he was able to give. So I will once again echo the sentiment—if you can, please give blood. If it wasn't for the generosity of strangers, she might not be lying beside me right now.

I kicked Andrew out of the room to try to get some sleep in the family lounge, and I have checked on him twice and he seems to be getting some sleep. I am glad, because tomorrow when they extubate her, we are going to need all outer strength, emotional and physical, to help her recover.

I did, however see her eyes slit open for a second, and she was kicking and flailing when the nurses moved her, so there is one big sigh of relief—all her bits work. :)

—Mom

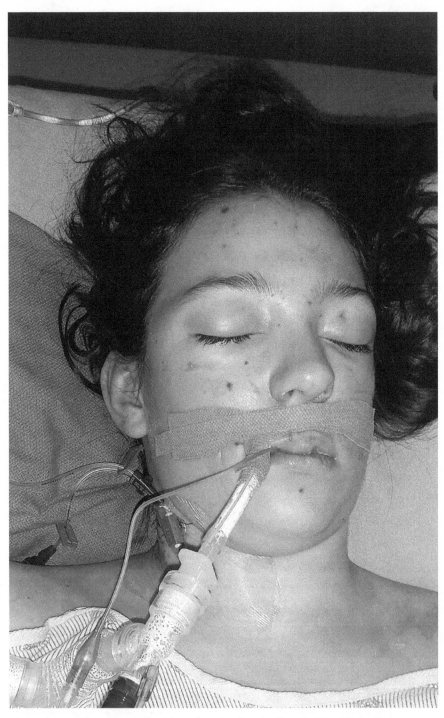

Avery, hours after surgery. Intubated and sedated. (Family Photo)

ANDREW: 24

January 21, 2015 (+11 Hours Post Op)

We've been at the hospital for 24 hours. Let me tell you that the first twelve hours were a cake walk compared to the twelve that came after and the twelve that are ahead.

Extubating happening this morning. Hopefully the fever is under control. Jodi stayed in the room and got a bit of sleep after a couple bouts of excitement. I grabbed a couple z's on some chairs. Princess Pants is strong and fighting. Some good kicks and resistance to the nurses (trying to keep her tube in).

No machines are beeping at the moment. This is a good thing. The sound of the ventilator overpowers the quiet room. I'm afraid to move and upset the Feng Shui.

Something just beeped and woke Jodi up. The nurse came in. One of the many bags of something feeding her medication was due for another dose. It was the sedative. They'll be waking her up soon.

I'm going to get a coffee and brush my teeth.

—Dad

EIGHT

HEALING

If you never have to see your child awakened from more than 24 hours of sedation, intubated, and in incredible pain then consider yourself fortunate. Also count your lucky stars if you never have to hear your child say, "Daddy, why am I hallucinating?" because as humorous as that sounds it means that they are being given some serious drugs to help manage some serious pain.

The job of the surgical team was complete. At this point the focus shifted to Avery and it was time for her to get busy making the best of all the work that had been done on her. Working with the nurses and support staff, Avery had a productive but rough couple days after surgery.

But first, we needed to get Avery up and remove the uncomfortable breathing tube from her throat.

By morning, Avery's hives had disappeared and some of the swelling in her face had gone down. There were a couple times when Avery woke up and started to flail but the nurses were quick to get her sedated again. On the upside it appeared that she had all her mobility and was good and strong. By nine o'clock in the morning the ICU team felt that it was time to wake Avery up but to do this they needed her as alert as possible and that meant there was be nothing in her system making her sleepy and there wasn't any pain medication.

I know what panic feels like. I've suffered with panic on and off for my entire adult life. However, it's not always clear to people on the outside what panic looks like. The moment they woke Avery up was not one of those times. Even with Jodi and I right at Avery's bedside, when she woke up you could see the panic in her eyes. Thankfully, the nurses had done this a thousand times before and made quick work of the procedure.

First, they explained to Avery that she needed to be untied, but only after she agreed to not try to take the tube out of her throat. Then, they gave Avery some instructions so the extubating would go as optimally as possible. Once the tube was out all Avery wanted was a glass of water but unfortunately that wasn't possible. There were rules and protocols that had to be followed. Having been denied a glass of water, panic quickly faded to pouting. It was at this point where I think I realized that things would soon be back to normal.

The first order of business was to get her morphine pump working. The instructions were very clear: Avery was the ONLY person who could hit the button. The device was set up so that it would only administer a certain amount of drug so Avery could press the button as often as she liked but she would only receive morphine as often as the machine was programmed to. The first hit sent her into la-la land in a hurry, which was good, because at this point we had a good handle on the full extent of her injuries.

After Avery gave herself a second hit she looked up at me and said, "Daddy, why am I hallucinating?" That's when I knew it was working. I explained to her that it was just the medicine keeping her comfortable and she smiled and closed her eyes.

Once Avery settled into her awake but drugged state we got a visit from a few doctors. I was lucky enough to speak to the surgical resident that worked with Dr. Missiuna in the operating room and he gave me the complete rundown of the surgery, and how it went better than expected and everyone involved did a wonderful job. He also informed me that Avery was the recipient of five litres of blood. In case you are wondering, because I sure was, that's about as much blood as a person has in their whole body. So, Avery came out of surgery without a drop of blood that she went in there with. A pint of it was mine.

The anesthesiologist came for a brief visit and explained his theory that it was the blood that caused the allergic reaction. My blood? We'll never know. What we do know is that the only reason Avery made it through the surgery as planned was because there was enough blood on hand from people's donations. I asked Canadian Blood Services on Twitter (@ItsInYouToGive) how many people I had to thank for giving the gift of life to Avery and their response was, depending on the situation, probably around fourteen people.

—

The day following Avery's awakening is a bit of a blur for me. Jodi sent me home to get some rest and visit with AJ, who was in fine form as you read at the very beginning of this story. Aside from that exchange all he wanted was to be reassured that Avery was okay and then cuddle with me on the couch.

I slept long and hard that first night back in my own bed. It was absolutely heaven. The setup at the hospital was quite a bit different but still better than what most people have to deal with. In the province of Ontario, Avery was guaranteed a ward room for her recovery. A ward room contains four beds. Because both Jodi and I have supplemental insurance through work, Avery was guaranteed a semi-private room for the duration of her stay. A semi-private room is two beds to a room. Upon inquiring about private room rates when we registered Avery the day before we were told that we only needed to pay the difference between our health coverage and the private rate, which worked out to something like $35 a day. Sold!

The private room had a chair that folded out into the most uncomfortable single bed I've ever slept in. There are also announcements and machines beeping and people moaning and crying all the time. It is a hospital after all, and a children's one at that. No one is there because everything is okay. Sleep is a rare commodity and I can't imagine how much less I would have gotten in a non-private room.

Now, Jodi and I are fortunate enough to live within a 45-minute drive from the hospital, and have a car, and supplemental health insurance, and have enough left over after bills are paid that we can afford some perks. So many families are not in that situation, and while our healthcare system will pay for all the necessities, it does not cover more than the basics. This is where Ronald McDonald House comes in.

Ronald McDonald House (RMH) provides a home away from home for families with children in hospital. There have been a couple mentions of it in this book so far and there are a couple more and that's because it is worth mentioning repeatedly. This is a charity that makes a direct and profound impact on the lives of families dealing with unimaginable health issues. As a parent who spent fifty percent of his time for the greater part of a week wedged in a hospital room and wandering the halls I can tell you that RMH makes a difference.

It wasn't until the second day at the hospital that I even realized that there was a Ronald McDonald House "family room" on our floor. I can't remember if it was Jodi who told me, or if I stumbled upon it during one of my wanderings, but there it was in all its glory. It was a room away from the hustle and bustle of the rest of the hospital. All you had to do was sign in and there were desks and couches, a couple TVs, and a kitchenette where you could make yourself a PB&J sandwich or toast a bagel. They even had muffins and soups and an assortment of beverages available. Most importantly, I think, was the fact that the only beeping you heard was the microwave.

Jodi and I leveraged this room quite a bit. Parents staying at the full RMH across the street used it as a go-between and a place to keep other family members occupied and relaxed. I used it so I wouldn't feel like I was living in a hospital. Avery used it in the sense that we could go get her some tea or a snack whenever the feeling struck.

—

The goals for Avery at this stage were pragmatic and tangible: eliminate the dependence on the pain medications, start eating and drinking and performing the corresponding bodily functions, get rid of the many tubes and wires, and get out of bed and walk.

In looking at the bandages that ran from the base of Avery's neck all the way down to her tailbone, it was near impossible for me to see how she was going to accomplish the walking. But, as you might know, kids have an amazing way of surprising you. It was in those first few days after surgery that I came to realize that I was the luckiest man in the world because I had a daughter who was also my hero (I told you there would be one).

Our son was also suitably amazed with everything, as evidenced in this exchange after I got home from the hospital after the surgery:

"Daddy, so Avery has screws and rods now?"

"Yes, she has two rods and twenty-seven screws."

"Are they on the outside or the inside?"

"They are on the inside."

"And they had to cut her open to get them in there?"

"Yes, they did."

"They sewed her back up though, right?"

ANDREW: SHE'S BACK!

January 21, 2015 (+20.5 Hours Post Op)

A lot has happened since the last update. From my perspective it was hell on Earth but according to the medical professionals it was business as usual.

Avery woke up and was trying to speak and pull the tube out of her throat. They sedated her again, but not for long. When the sedative wore off it was time to remove the breathing tube. Holding her hands down and watching her struggle to breathe is now rightfully at the top of my list of moments I'd rather not have to experience again.

The good news is she was telling us to let go of her hands and sit her up and get her some water. Unfortunately we were unable to do two of the three at that moment but after about an hour we had her sitting up and breathing normally. The smile she gave the nurse who hooked her up to the pain meds pump was priceless!

I spoke to the resident who assisted Dr. Missiuna. They are very happy with how it all went. She's fused from T2 to L4, which totals 14 vertebrae. She has two rods holding her spine rigid but in an optimal posture. Holding the rods in are 27 screws, cemented into place. Why not 28 (14 x 2)? Her T4 wasn't well suited for a screw so they skipped it on the one side. Both Dr. Missiuna and the resident are happy with it. They transfused her two times throughout the surgery, using my blood and then a whack of blood bank blood. This was due to natural processes and the sheer length of the surgery. She was never in any danger.

She's sitting in a chair now and reasonably comfortable. Nurse Janet is very impressed. She continues to be ahead of the curve. We need to make sure she's taking big deep breaths to stave off fluid build-up in her lungs. We do exercises with a special machine every hour.

As it stands she's the healthiest kid in the ICU and the beds are full so if they need her bed they will move her into an interim care room and then a ward room. I know it's all good news but having Nurse Janet right outside the window is a great comfort.

As of 2:30 PM Avery was back lying down and overachieving in every category. She burped and that was a big deal so they gave her a popsicle (mango, her favourite) and she immediately started talking better. She was also allowed some water. The hard part is going to be slowing her down! She wants to do everything she can and we have to remind her to let the nurses do the work and she needs to just relax. Such a fighter.

Jodi slept not too badly and will likely sleep not too badly tonight so Avery said it was okay if I went home and got some rest and saw The Dude. I'll relieve Jodi on the day shift tomorrow. All things considered things are going as expected now in spite of the rocky night and rough morning.

My brain is mush, so hopefully this update made some sense. I'm going to take a nap.

—Dad

JODI: WHAT A DIFFERENCE A DAY MAKES
January 21, 2015 (+24 Hours Post Op)

I am not sure I even have the words for the difference between now and 24 hours ago—or for that matter, even nine hours ago. Watching Avery healing with such ease and grace has just lifted a world of worry off my shoulders. As late as 9:30 AM this morning she was still intubated and hysterical any time she came to (understandably). Her eyes were swollen shut and she had so many IVs in.

Now, she can talk—almost audibly, eat and roll from side to side. She watched a movie and decided it was time for bed—I may soon join her as I am spent and I doubt it will be a truly restful night.

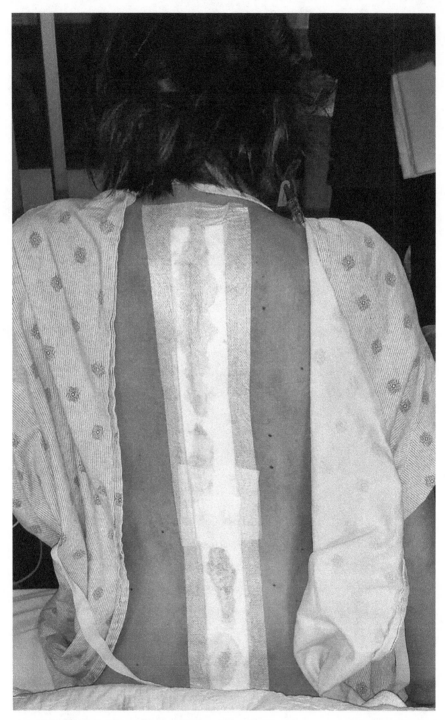

Avery's incision held together with tape. (Family Photo)

I wandered in to the Ronald McDonald House room on this floor—free coffee and snacks until 11:00 PM. Colonel Sanders adorns the wall outside of 3B and in the hall one of the wings is sponsored by Walmart.

And lastly for tonight's ramblings, the hospital is selling a stuffed something and neither Andrew nor I were certain what it is—possibly a pig with horse legs. :)

Thanks for hanging in here with us. I don't think we can articulate how much your collective support has helped us get through these last 36 hours.

—Mom

JODI: DAY 2 UPDATE
January 22, 2015 (Post Op Day 2)

Avery has taken up court in the paediatric wing and seems to be settling in. Day 2 pain is a little higher than day 1, but they have also taken off the continuous release med, so for pain she is relying on her pump.

The physiotherapist had her sitting in a chair, but she was done with that after about an hour and honestly looked uncomfortable the whole time. We figure her organs are settling in their new and proper homes, and that is making her not feel so great. The nurse cleared her for a Jolly Rancher hard candy, so that has been her primary sustenance. The kitchen offered her some toast and peanut butter—she was excited about that, and did manage to eat almost a third of the piece.

Today she doesn't want to be up, preferring to recline at about 20°. The tape on her chest is making her itchy, but not the worst. They removed one of her IV lines this morning, and we are hopeful to have either the central line in her neck or the remaining inactive line in her right hand removed today too.

Andrew has decided that he wants to stay tonight—I really think she would be fine on her own, but maybe Andrew needs this for him—but after a night of constant alarms and nurses, he may decide that we are better for her when we are rested.

I noted that her right leg, which was sitting at about one centimetre shorter than the left before surgery, appeared even shorter when I looked at *her lying in bed, but admittedly she wasn't lying straight, so hopefully it was just how she was positioned.*

I saw the surgical resident who aided in the surgery and he told me he was fairly certain I was mistaken, but until she is steady enough for x-rays, I will just have to trust him.

I stepped outside for a few minutes this morning, realising I hadn't breathed fresh air since early Tuesday. Hopefully Avery will be a little more mobile tomorrow—or they will allow her to go in a wheelchair so we can walk around a little.

Oh, Avery's question for today was how much do the rods weigh? Surgical resident figured less than a pound.

—Mom

ANDREW: TALES FROM THE WARD
January 22, 2015 (Post Op Day 2)

So Jodi sent me home yesterday afternoon. I got home about thirty seconds before grandpa came home with The Dude and he was thrilled to see me. Unfortunately I was beyond exhausted and only got to spend a few minutes with him before crashing. I managed to get up and go with him to bowling practice, so that was nice.

After a pretty good sleep I checked in with Jodi to see how our superstar princess was doing. She slept but nurses come in every couple hours to poke and prod so her sleep is fragmented. Jodi didn't sleep much as there are alarms that go off constantly and just a lot of activity on the floor in general. I'm back at the hospital now and Dude is coming to visit with grandpa after school. Jodi will go back with him and I'll be staying here.

They stopped her background pain meds (a constant stream to supplement the morphine pump) so it's just the pump now. I don't see her hammering the pump button all the time; it's usually lit for a while before she hits it, so that's good.

She just rolled over onto her side, mostly on her own. I can tell she's not super comfortable but she's calm and relaxing reasonably well so that's good. Just waiting for another visit from the physiotherapist and the nurse (on her regular rotation).

Not a very exciting update, but honestly, I'd be perfectly okay with only posting ones like these from now on.

—Dad

ANDREW: QUESTION PERIOD
January 22, 2015 (Post Op Day 2)

Day 2 in the books and we take some questions.

Jodi has made her way home after a short visit from The Dude and grandpa. Pants wasn't too alert but did manage a couple smiles. Dr. Missiuna came by when I was down at dinner and said that she was still ahead of where they expected her to be. That's good news but she's still in a lot of discomfort and just wants to go home.

She's due for vitals check and more pain meds at 8:00. The nurses will be by at 12:00, 4:00, and 8:00 and Jodi will be back sometime before 10:00 AM. Hopefully we can get her up tomorrow as she only spent about an hour sitting upright today.

The night nurse just came in and discovered that her left arm was experiencing infiltration. That's where the IV leaks into the arm instead of the vein. It was all swollen and tight. Also, not all her meds from the pump were getting into her system. The nurse switched the lines to her right arm and took out the IV from the left arm completely and Pants's mood improved immediately. Hopefully at some point tonight they'll take out her main line—the one that goes into her neck. Fewer tubes is good news.

Now for some questions from the press gallery:

- *Will they ever remove the hardware in her spine?*

- *Will she still grow?*

- *If so, do they adjust the hardware?*

The short answers are "no," "yes," "no."

It's much too risky to have to open her up again and unscrew the rods. It's a terribly invasive surgery that involves the spinal column so once they're done with the installation they leave it there forever. There are cases where they have been removed but this is very rare. As for growth, she is growing in two places: her legs (femurs) and her spine. Fortunately, due to her age and physical development she does not have too much spinal growth remaining (the second opinion doc at Sick Kids estimated a couple centimetres).

The area that's fused is 14 vertebrae and there will not be any further growth. As such, the hardware will stay the way it is and her vertebrae will fuse together and that's the spine she'll have for the rest of her days. I have got to tell you though, from what I've seen to this point it's mighty fine-looking. Such an improvement over the crooked, asymmetrical one she had before! Now, it's possible she may realize some growth from the remaining vertebrae but it will not be significant. She will still grow in her legs though so she's not done getting taller quite yet.

*If anyone has any other questions just leave a comment or send us a message on Facebook or via email **bentbutnotbrokencanada@gmail.com***

—Dad

ANDREW: QUOTES AND SATS
January 22, 2015 (Post Op Day 2)

"I want to go home. Why can't I just go home?"

"I wish I could live a different life until all this was over."

"Why is everyone asking me to hurt myself?"

These are all things that Pants said to me over the last 8 hours, the last one just before midnight. Her oxygen saturation levels were dipping below 90 even though she was breathing just fine (95 or better is what we want to see). The nurse was asking her to cough and take deep breaths and that makes her back hurt. I was getting her to breathe deeply and her levels were getting up into the 90s again but would dip back down after she stopped the deep inhalations. Apparently this is common when kids (and possibly adults) are on morphine and sleeping deeply. At least that's what the nurse told me. I Googled it and didn't get the search terms right I'm sure because all I found were links to terrifying studies I could have gone all week without having seen.

Stupid Internet.

The nurse went away and came back with a cylindrical container of water that she attached to the oxygen hole in the wall and then hooked up one of those over-the-ear and up-your-nose plastic tubes. Immediately her SATs spiked back. The oxygen bong was working!

Pants said to me, "I feel like Hazel Grace," I asked her if that was April Grace's mother or grandmother and Pants made a face; one of sheer disappointment that, had she been in a healthier mood, would have come with a "Dad-dy!" (if you know my daughter you have heard this many times before). She then informed me that Hazel was the terminally ill kid from The Fault in Our Stars. *I made sure she knew that this was a little different and that she didn't have cancer, she just had morphine. She hit her button and gave me her best smile. That kid has got impeccable comedic timing.*

All was well again. Also, they are performing maintenance on the code red system, so if you have a code red, dial extension 5555—or get in touch with Colonel Jessup.

To wrap up the evening's midnight festivities she closed with a quote that would make Charlie Sheen proud:

"I just took five pills!" [All at once]

drops mic

—Dad

NINE

PASSING THE TESTS

After the first couple of days things really get moving in both the figurative and literal sense. Beds on a paediatric ward are at a premium, but the good news was Avery didn't require much attention from the nurses. More importantly, a large part of the healing process was for Avery to learn how to move her new body around.

The timetable for days three to seven were set from the beginning, with Day 3 consisting of walking and Day 7 being her last day in the hospital. In between, there would be the removal of all her tubes and wires, more walking, x-rays, more walking, and finally some more walking and a flight of stairs!

This was the most exciting time for everyone because it was known at this point that everything was as it should be and it was now a matter of Avery putting in the time and working on the instructions given to her by the hospital-assigned physiotherapist.

This was also a hard time for me because I had to go back to work on the Monday. I would get to go pick Avery and Jodi up from the hospital Tuesday afternoon, but it marked the longest stretch of time since the surgery that I was away from her. Because of this, I took a few night shifts in a row at the hospital. It was... interesting, to say the least.

First of all, as previously mentioned, the ward was filled with children with varying ailments, and with those ailments came a varying number of visits from the nursing staff. This meant that there was no rhyme or reason to when I was awakened by some machine or upset child.

Secondly, I got a really good idea of how the hospital used its paging system. That is to say, it didn't matter what time it was, if the page was important enough it would be repeated over and over and over again.

Lastly, I would be remiss if I didn't sing the praises of the nursing and support staff at this point. They worked long, tireless hours doing a lot of unglamorous jobs. They not only had to care for the children but they also had to care for the parents. I tried my best not to be a burden and not ask for too many things or ask too many unnecessary questions. They were, after all, there to provide care to a number of sick and scared children and not act as Nurse Google for a curious parent.

It was during the three long nights I spent in ward 3B that one nurse stood out from the rest. I don't even remember her name, and for that I feel terrible, because she was in a class all her own and deserves to be recognized. Maybe it is best that she remain nameless for this book to avoid any sort of awkwardness at work, but she was truly amazing, both in caring for Avery and in making sure I was taken care of, too.

Here's a tip for you: write down the names of everyone you want to thank. I'm not certain I can track everyone's name down so they can receive their proper accolades and it would have been better to just write it all down at the time.

—

I had the privilege of spending nights two through five at the hospital and it wasn't long before time had no meaning. The trade-off was the progress Avery was making and seeing her when she was rested and alert, before the trials of the day drained her energy reserves. Also, and maybe it's a parental thing, but seeing your child in a peaceful slumber is one of the greatest things in the world.

I can remember the days of paranoid parenting and checking in on my sleeping baby what seemed like every fifteen minutes. That soon changed to checking on her simply because I had never cared for anyone else in my life nearly this much and seeing Avery asleep became a moment of quiet reflection.

It was nice to have a few of those moments over the course of five nights—in between all the interruptions and beeping and announcements over the communications system, that is.

The goal was to bust Avery out of that joint on Day 7 of post op, with me going to work for the Monday morning before that. In order for that to happen, Avery had to pass several tests: functioning without any tubes or IVs in her, eating, drinking, walking, and climbing stairs. There may have been a few more things on the discharge checklist but those were the ones I remember the most.

Avery being Avery went and did everything pretty much exactly on schedule and at a level considered to be quite high. Such an overachiever!

The one that brought me to tears, however, was the first time since the surgery that she walked.

ANDREW: SHE WALKS!

January 23, 2015 (Post Op Day 3)

We have had a great night / morning. Pants woke me up a few times asking for water and only gave me minimal grief when I said she had to sleep instead of watching TV.

When morning finally came she was feeling good and ate a whole apple and finished her apple juice. The first substantial amount of real food she's eaten since Monday night (though she did manage 1/3 of a piece of peanut butter toast yesterday).

The physiotherapist came by at 9:00 AM and Avery was still digesting so she asked that she come back in half an hour. When she returned we took a few minutes to get Avery standing up and then it was out into the hallway with her. She walked out about eight feet and then walked about six feet back and has been sitting in a chair for almost two hours now. She's positively exhausted from such a busy morning.

Her whole class video-called shortly after her journey to the hallway and back and when they all heard she had taken her first steps they erupted into applause and cheering. Brought tears to my eyes.

She's resting now and we're just keeping an eye on her abdomen. The

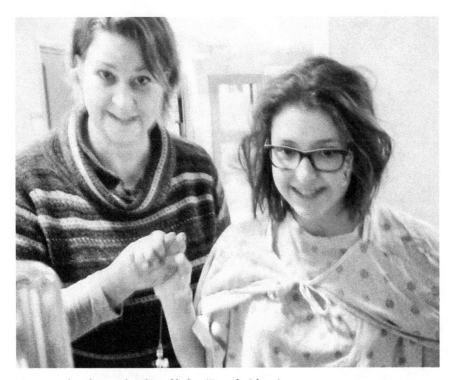

Avery on her feet with a bit of help. (Family Photo)

drugs work a number on the GI system and we want to make sure everything is okay there. Hopefully the neck IV comes out today too.

That's it for the morning of Day 3 of post op. I have lost all sense of time.

—Dad

JODI: PROGRESS

January 23, 2015 (Post Op Day 3)

It truly amazes me the progress Avery has made in these past three days! Today Avery added walking to her list of accomplishments post-surgery. After she was done with the walking and settled back down, she said the walking didn't bother her at all, but the getting up to walking and the sitting back down afterwards hurts—and that hurt scares her, so she doesn't really want to do it. And I feel like perhaps we have different motivations for this, so I will need to rethink my encouragements.

Pre-surgery we had explained that in order for her to come home she needed to eat, poop, and walk. Post-surgery we have added the interim step of the removal of the catheter and all her lines including her pain pump in the pre-pooping stage. Today she said she didn't really want the catheter out because then she would have to get up and walk to the washroom ... so I need a better sell.

I was excited when I got here today to hear that she ate a whole apple. Lunch didn't go over as well with all the walking and sitting in a chair for three hours, but I held out some hope for dinner. Aunt Kari showed up mid-afternoon with the promised snuck-in mint chocolate chip ice cream from Baskin-Robbins, which Avery gratefully accepted. She managed to eat a tablespoon or so of that then needed a rest.

One of the excellent staff came by to see what she wanted for dinner—the Friday night special being meatloaf with mashed potatoes and peas—she wasn't interested in the meatloaf, but asked for the potatoes—with gravy—and a bowl of soup and some apple slices. This was apparently a very odd dinner order, as the guy who brought up the tray called me to make sure this was actually what she wanted. She ate a tablespoon of potatoes and a spoonful of soup then pushed the tray away. I think she is starting to get the link between food and poop.

She has been drinking tea. Maybe not the ideal beverage for a twelve-year-old, but on the beer scale of urine colours, she is clearly sufficiently hydrated.

The video chat with her class did her wonders, and the cheers and applause when she announced she walked was amazing—I think Andrew said it brought a tear to his eye, well it did to mine too (mind you when I stalked by one of her friend's house this morning to pass on that it would be nice if they could call her again today, I had a tear then, too). She really has some awesome friends. Her teacher is hoping to make it up for a visit, if not Sunday then early next week, and around dinner her Principal called to see how she was doing.

Andrew said she had been consistent with her pain pump for the first two days at about 200 hits each day, and unless something goes south later today, I am certain that number will be significantly less tomorrow—which also heads us the right direction to transition her to oral pain meds and losing yet another line.

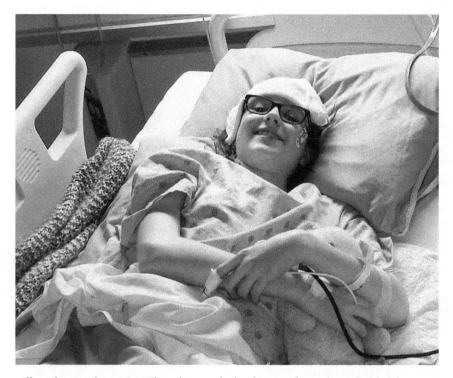

All smiles watching TV… though it might be the morphine. (Family Photo)

Andrew and I just moved her bed so she could still watch TV while she is on her side—I hope the nurses aren't upset.

:) Thanks for following!

—Mom

ANDREW: OLD SCHOOL BATMAN THEME SONG
January 24, 2015 (Post-op Night 3 / Day 4)

Last night the nurse was wearing a Batman t-shirt. She's been my favourite so far :) Avery took her Tylenol and long acting oral pain meds (only three pills) and then hit her morphine pump. A couple minutes later she started talking in her sleep, "When's the next course?"

"Four hours sweetie. Batman will be back in four hours."

I had a dream that a couple friends had me over for dinner and instead of offering me a regular bottle of wine they took out this wine bottle that had a peel backside. They lay it down on the counter, took a bread knife out

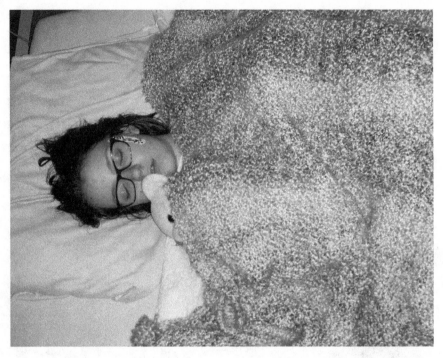

Sleeping princess. (Family Photo)

and slid it through this lengthwise opening, and cut me off a slice of fish. I think it was a Northern Pike Grigio.

Now I'm beginning to wonder if maybe Batnurse wasn't slipping me some of the good meds in the water she brought for me.

Pants had a rough night.

She couldn't get comfortable. Also, one of her IVs was leaking (down her arm this time, not into her arm) so she probably wasn't getting her full dose when she hit the PCA button. They got her IV switched over this morning and hopefully that will improve things. We need her to hit the machine less so she can transition to oral meds—a requirement for going home—but she needs to also manage the pain so she can do her physio. It's a balancing act that she hasn't quite figured out yet.

Today we are going to focus on getting her eating more and walking more. The surgical resident figures she'll be standing on her own comfortably enough by Monday so they can take some X-rays. Her goal for today is to

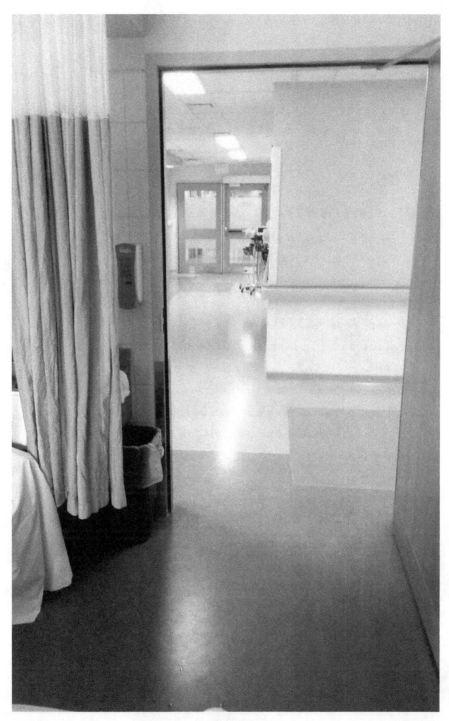

The long walk to the bathroom. (Family Photo)

get up and walk twice and by the end of the second trip travel almost three times farther than she did yesterday.

Aunt Stacey will visit too with a possible appearance from The Dude (who misses his big sister) so it's going to be a full day.

Jodi's going to tag me out after The Dude's bowling and I'll go home and get some proper rest before coming back later tonight.

—Dad

JODI: TIME WARP

January 24, 2015 (Post Op Day 4)

Day 4? What time is it? Where are we?

Another eventful day at McMaster. Avery showed her stubborn side this morning by refusing to do her physio until I got here, even though she knew that would be after 1:00 PM.

As not to totally embarrass her, let's just say she checked off one of the three things she needed to do to be able to go home off that list :)

The physiotherapist arrived around 2:30 PM and we had already gotten the room all prepared so as not to waste any more of her time. Avery was entirely bewildered about how it was she was supposed to get from lying to standing, but after a little refresher got to upright. She walked twice as far as she did yesterday and even a little faster. She'll be scooting down that hallway in no time. And Andrew and I were cleared to be her hall shuffling escorts—so if he is back tonight perhaps we will try to get that second walk in after all.

Since she was feeling a little flushed, we just did up her gown instead of adding the robe today—which only sucked for the entire time she was sitting as I hadn't been quick enough to untie the back and she found it terribly restrictive to sit in.

While she was in the chair I wiped down her legs, I guess that is almost a bath. After just under an hour, she was so uncomfortable she felt she needed back in bed. We did manage to get her some fresh sheets and a clean gown. I hope we are getting closer to losing some of her tubes and lines, but have decided asking doesn't really do much for us.

I was quite pleased when Avery ordered the fish sticks for dinner—and when they came she even ate 1.5 of them. Protein for the win!

Otherwise, it seems Pants keeps herself quite cool so the finger monitor keeps not being able to get a proper read. The one nurse was going to try a toe, but then felt her ice-brick feet and immediately went to find a heated blanket to wrap around her toes.

So now we wait for Pants's wishes for the night. Andrew is planning on coming back, and I promised the PT I would be back by 9:00 AM, but we'll see. Sometimes a girl just wants her (less snoring) mother as her roommate.

If anything else exciting happens, we'll be sure to post.

—Mom

ANDREW: SUPER MARIO THEME SONG
January 25, 2015 (Post Op Day 5)

Batnurse was assigned to Avery again last night but she had on a different t-shirt. This time she was Super Mario!

Avery had a rough night. She couldn't get comfortable and was complaining quite a bit. She did manage to doze off a couple times but I think I slept more than she did. There's a baby on the floor now and let's just say the poor thing has one hell of a set of lungs.

She is attempting to eat breakfast because she knows today will be a big day and she's going to need her energy. We're going for a couple walks and will extend her range past the hallway corner and hopefully to the bathroom!

The pain doctors were here and suggested Pants stop using the pump and instead switch to a combination of short term (four hour) and long term (eight hour) hydromorphone pills with Tylenol by request.

—

So the weekend PT came before I could post this and much has transpired. Pants walked all the way to the bathroom! She spent some time freshening up and looks like a whole new person.

Not one to settle for one stretch goal she decided to kick things into high gear and make the walk back with nothing to support her but her IV pole and the PT's hand—and the PT says she was barely using it!

She's resting in a chair now as we await the surgeon to remove the main-line in her neck as well as a whole whack of tubes.

She was granted anything she wanted as a reward for her spectacular efforts today. Her choice? A glass of water, some silly television, and to be left alone for some peace and quiet!

Have we told you how much we love this kid?

—Dad

JODI: NO STRINGS ATTACHED
January 25, 2015 (Post Op Day 5)

What an amazing day! I arrived at the hospital shortly after 9:00 and Avery was still munching on her fruit loops and banana for breakfast. Lisa, the physiotherapist arrived around 10:00 and Avery was pretty quick to get to standing and walked down the hall right to the washroom.

While she took a seat and tried to relax a little, we took advantage of the sink and towels and cleaned her up a bit for her first non-family visitors. The walk back she pushed her IV pole and only held Lisa's hand for comfort more than support, then turned herself and sat down without any help (well aside from me opening the back of her gown—she is very hot with ice-brick extremities).

She stayed sitting for over an hour, briefly spoke with her visitors then got back to standing with little assistance and back to bed. Her IV was bothering her, so after a few complaints her nurse removed it—and didn't replace it! She said she would wait until the resident showed up, unless Avery started peeing much darker than Coors Light.

Her room gets lovely daytime sun, but as a result, her room gets wickedly hot while the sun is up, then cools off fast when the sun sets. Pants's mannerisms remind me of me when I was having her—hot and not wanting anything on me and no one to speak to me.

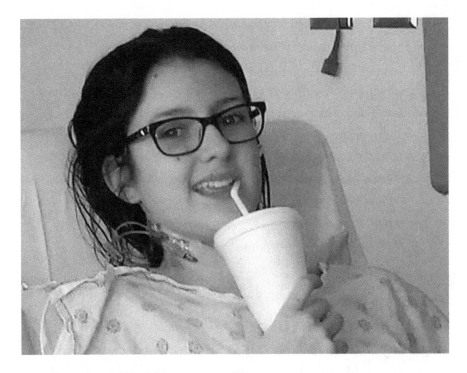

She smiles! (Family Photo)

Then she ate lunch 2.3 fish sticks, some carrots and one Dad's oatmeal cookie. She needed a little rest, but at 2:00 asked me to take her to the washroom again, so since dad was gone, we called over Nurse Sandy and trekked down the hall—me with her catheter bag hanging off my jean pocket as she no longer had her IV pole to hang it from. She walked back that time all by herself—me trailing a step behind with the pee bag. She got herself seated with no help and watched some TV. I needed to grab some lunch and left for about ten minutes, and noted her room was on the call board when I re-entered the floor so I hurried back in. Seems she wanted back in bed—so we just did that—she used her awesome squat muscles and pushed up to standing then sat on her bed and lay down—all by herself.

Around 4:00 her surgeon showed up (and scared the pants off Nurse Sandy!) and ordered the central line out—but then volunteered to do it himself. Seems that one gets stitched in to place, so he removed the stitches and left the nurse to bandage it. He also told her she could remove the catheter.

So by 4:30 she was officially line and tube free and can roam as she wishes. She does have to pee in a 'hat' to measure her outputs, but that is nothing.

Oh—and in case you didn't know already, the patient services at this hospital are amazing. We were invited to a toy giveaway at 2:00. I figured McDonald's toys—but no, these were full-size toys. Colour explosion kits, trucks, dolls, colouring sets—and all the name brand ones. Free. Just for being here. She didn't feel up for the walk, and I was going by around 3:00 when they were leaving and was called over to see if there was something she might like.

I anticipate a couple more walks tonight, then x-rays tomorrow and more physio with Jill and maybe bringing Pants home by Tuesday.

So here is Pants—no strings—wires or tubes—attached :)

—Mom

JODI: ALL FLUSHED OUT
January 26, 2015 (Post Op Day 6)

Just a quick update from evil night 6 on 3B. Avery found it impossible to get comfortable in her bed, and just when she would settle down, the urge to pee would hit—like every 97 minutes—so we'd get up to take care of that, then spend 80 minutes getting comfortable... you get the idea.

At 4:00 she thought I was sleeping too soundly, so she decided to just go to the bathroom by herself. Like got out of bed, slippers on, all by herself. Unfortunately for her, she dropped her gown on the floor and I jumped up to find a nearly naked Pants standing there. That wake-up worked out as she was due for the four-hour pain meds, and I had asked that if she was sleeping to skip that dose.

So far this morning (let's say morning started around 7:00) she has been down the hall to the washroom three times, nibbled some breakfast, sat in her chair for an hour and is back in bed waiting on the physiotherapist and x-rays.

I am still holding out for a nap, so my uber-comfortable hospital cot is still in bed form (it converts from a chair).

—Mom

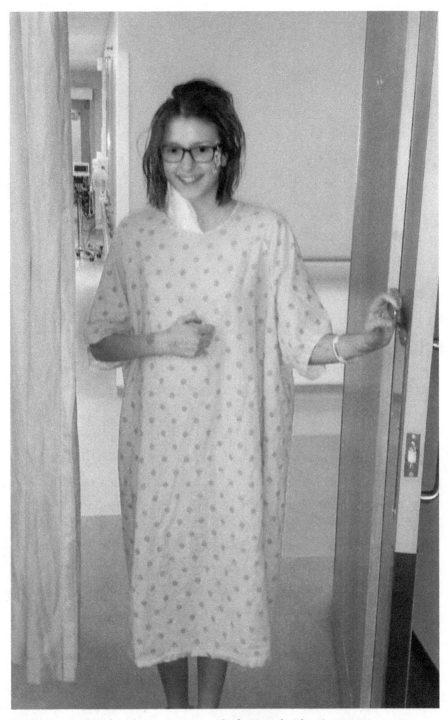

Walking unassisted with no strings attached. (Family Photo)

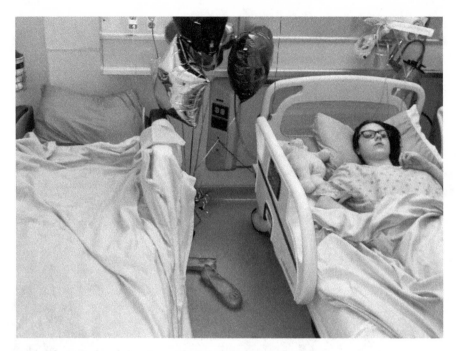

Not a five star hotel, but it got the job done. (Family Photo)

JODI: CLIMBING STAIRS LIKE A BOSS
January 26, 2015 (Post Op Day 6)

Another productive day, though without a clear release order for tomorrow, but we are optimistic it will work out that way. The resident who was by today said physio just had to clear her, to which I replied that after she sprinted up and down the stairs, physio said they don't need to see her again, so I took that as cleared. The steady flow of pee has finally tapered off as the last of the surgery/ IV fluid build-up has been passed, so we are at a much better walk frequency.

She still has no appetite, but tries to eat something each meal—I didn't even question her when she spit out the 'grilled chicken thigh' as it must have tasted like it smelled—so she agreed to some Froot Loops instead. I would love to see her actually eat like she is hungry, but right now she finds the effort of sitting up and moving food from tray to mouth exhausting. There is always tomorrow.

The other accomplishment for today was leaving the ward on her own feet to the playroom and back—without stopping as she didn't think the chairs looked too comfortable.

So I think we just need some x-rays and then we can leave, but apparently there is a process to that and it hasn't happened yet. We get asked by lots of people about the release plans and have to say we don't know. Maybe I will just tell them we are leaving tomorrow and see what happens.

Here's to hopefully a more restful sleep for both of us.

—Mom

JODI: LAST HOSPITAL DAY :)

January 27, 2015 (Post Op Day 7)

Night 7 was by far the best one so far. Pants fell asleep before 9:00 and woke up around midnight for a bathroom trip—but this again worked out as midnight is a med round. She fell almost immediately back to sleep and woke up again around 3:30 for a quick trip down the hall, then climbed right back in to bed and was asleep again before I had her covers pulled up. She slept until 6:30 and then decided it was morning.

I had a tepid shower in the family shower unit. Refreshing!

X-rays have been completed—though Pants really did not like the process, mostly because the wheelchair did not support her head and that made it hard for her to focus. I stood behind her for a bit and let her lie her greasy hair on my belly. The orderly was taking too long so I brought her back up to the ward by myself. We walked past the main entrance and she was quite happy to feel the breeze coming through the doors. Her new nurse has said there is some sort of hair-washing apparatus that can be brought in, so hopefully we can get that taken care of as she is still another week away from being allowed to shower.

Andrew is getting the house set up—we think the La-Z-Boy on the main floor is our best interim solution, though for the past two days she has preferred to be flat on her back. The fireplace living room gets some normal TV plus the Netflix so it maximizes her watching options and is beside the kitchen.

So now we wait. Hair wash, doctor visit and release orders. Next update from home. :)

—Mom

TEN

HOME SWEET HOME

It wasn't long before I started referencing how long Avery had been home instead of how long it had been since the surgery. In this book I stopped after one month, but when someone asked me how Avery was doing (which happened several times a day) it was only a week or so before I started responding with, "Great! She's been home for X days now and she's ahead of the curve in every category."

I used the expression "ahead of the curve" a lot on purpose to see if anyone would get the joke. Very few people did. The first few weeks that Avery was home were the times when people had the most questions. It's not like I was quiet about the surgery. Everyone I knew was aware of what was going on, but people were more interactive once they knew that Avery was home, recovering, and feeling better.

This was also the time when I witnessed firsthand how many kind people there were in my life. Everyone I interacted with who knew what Avery had just gone through took time out of their day to ask how she was doing and ask if there was anything the family needed. I have never felt as loved as a person as I did in the weeks and months that followed Avery's surgery.

—

There were goals for Avery when she was at home. First and foremost, she

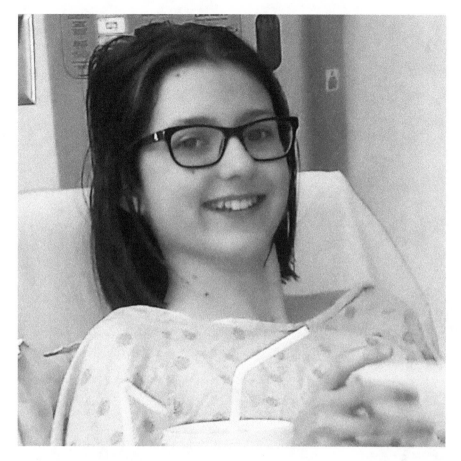

Feeling good. (Family Photo)

was to get her appetite back. Because Avery had been under general anesthetic for so long, it was expected that it would take about a month before she returned to normal in that department.

Another milestone that everyone at home was watching for was when she would pick up a book again. Avery was and still is a voracious reader so to see her without a book in her hand was particularly concerning. I am pleased to report that the reading bug did return, but it took a lot longer than I thought it would.

Then, there was this business about the scar. Obviously, there was infection to worry about. There always is with an open wound, and Avery had one hell of an open wound. As you saw in a photo from a blog post of Jodi's, Avery had

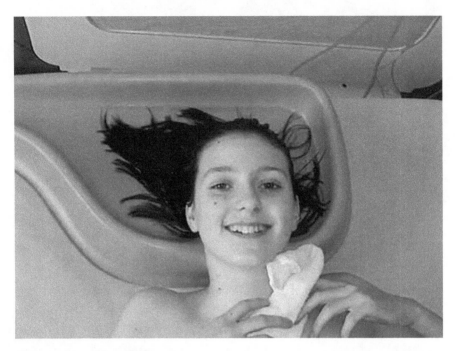

Hair washing. (Family Photo)

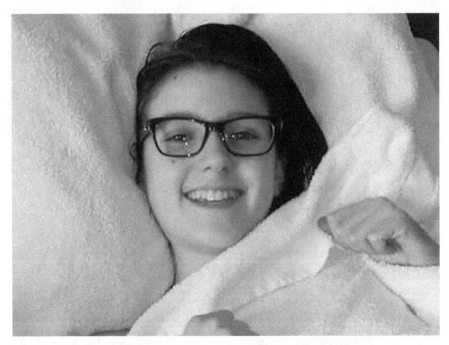

All cleaned up and ready to go home .(Family Photo)

Steri-Strips from the base of her neck down to the small of her back. At some point those strips would fall off and Avery would be left with what looked like a zipper running down her entire back.

One of the things that caused Avery to cry prior to the surgery was the thought that she would have this nasty scar on her back for the rest of her life. Which was understandable. If I was a pre-teen kid I'd be worried about my physical appearance too. Hell, I'm a grown adult and still have hang ups about some of my physical traits. So, there was some natural concern that when the strips started to fall off there would be an emotional outburst.

There was definitely an emotional outburst, only it was a positive one. Avery got a glimpse of her scar in the mirror once a few of the strips fell off and she loved it. Sometimes the only way to get through a difficult time is to own it and Avery was owning it like a boss. After all I had seen her go through over the weeks and months that preceded surgery, and after all the days and hours since they removed her breathing tube, Avery always found a way to surprise me with her strength.

Certainly, Avery was drawing some of that strength from her classmates. Seventh grade can be a tricky one and Jodi and I noticed that this was the time when the kids were splintering off into little cliques. We were very pleased with the friends Avery was closest with but there were definitely a few other girls in her class that didn't exactly give us warm fuzzy feelings. When it came to Avery's surgery, though, every single kid in her class showed tremendous amounts of support. It was one of the most heartwarming things I've ever seen.

So, a big goal for Avery over her initial recovery time was returning to school. Dr. Missiuna set a goal of returning to school for half an hour a day starting about a month following surgery. It took about that long for all the anaesthetic to work though her system and return Avery to normal. From there, the time away from home was increased slowly, about thirty minutes every week, until Avery was back in school full time. It was a long, slow process and it tested the patience of everyone involved, especially Avery who was used to everything happening quickly and with minimal effort. I'm the same way, but I have a few decades of experience in the disappointment department.

JODI: HOME AGAIN, HOME AGAIN, JIGGITTY-JIG

January 27, 2015 (Post Op Day 7, Going Home)

What a day! As we readied ourselves to go home, one of the nurses found us a lying hair wash thing, so I washed her hair.

Pants felt like a new person once she was cleaned up.

About an hour later, we were cleared to leave—conveniently at about the exact moment Andrew arrived, so Andrew gathered all our stuff and packed the car, and Pants put on some pants so we could go home.

he drive home was uneventful, and Pants was eager to get home. Once in the house, she took up court in the living room and asked for a toaster grilled cheese. I whipped that up for her and then she ate the whole thing! That is the most food I have seen her eat in a week!

I went out to fill her prescriptions and pick up the Dude—who was leaving school with one of Pants's best friends, so I brought her home for a quick visit. It was quite exciting to see Avery awake and engaged for the whole visit—leaps ahead of two days ago!

While I was out, Andrew managed to measure her:

Yep, 5.5 cm or 2.25 inches taller!

She requested food that doesn't need utensils for dinner, so we are going to try pulled pork sandwiches.

Next visit to the surgeon is on Friday, so we'll update later.

—Mom

ANDREW: TEN DAYS, TWO INCHES

January 28, 2015 (Post Op Day 8, 1 Day Home)

I went back to the office on Monday so that's why you've seen so many posts from Jodi over the last while. Jodi's taken a leave of absence to stay home with Pants for the next month while she recovers. I get to work. So it goes.

I don't have a whole lot new to update you with except to say that Princess Pants continues to exceed every expectation. She's walking with a bit more confidence every time she goes for a stroll or up and down the stairs. She can

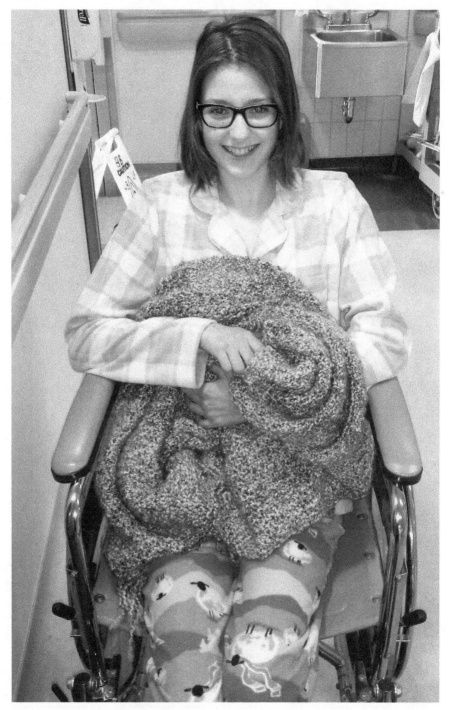

Let's roll! (Family Photo)

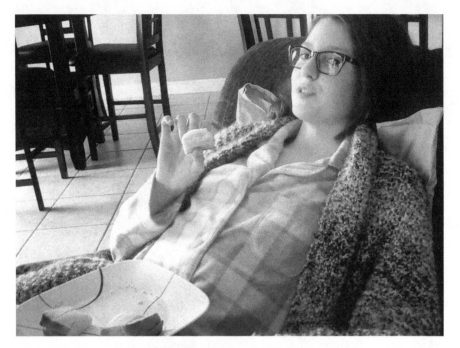

Home sweet home... and grilled cheese. (Family Photo)

get in and out of bed on her own. Even her appetite is returning, albeit slowly.

Avery promises to write a post soon to let you all in on the events of the past week from her perspective. Please be patient as pretty much everything she does is exhausting and typing out a big post will drain her.

In the meantime, I took some before and after photos and put them together side by side so you could get an idea of the difference. I flipped the before picture so the lines would line up a bit better so imagine her bent the other direction for the pic on the left. Also, this is far from precise. I didn't get the angles and distances quite right so the proportions weren't perfect. Nevertheless you get a really good idea of the difference.

Left: Before surgery (Jan. 18). Right: After surgery (Jan. 28)

For those who many not have seen it in a previous post the difference in height is 5.5 cm (or roughly 2 1/4 inches). Pants now stands at an impressive 168.3 cm (5' 6.25").

—Dad

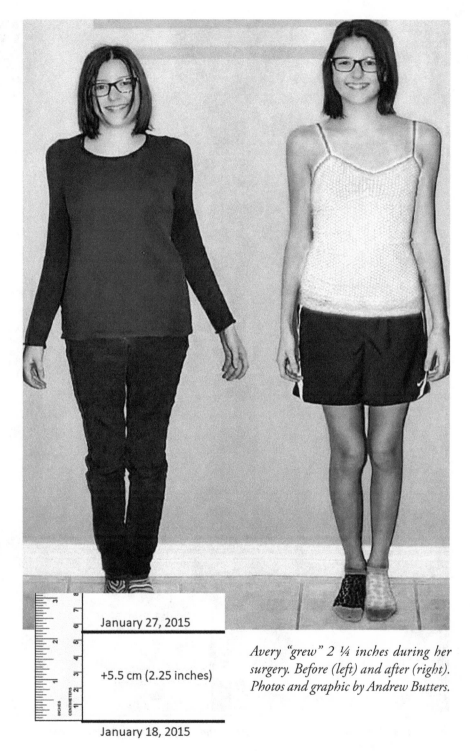

January 27, 2015

+5.5 cm (2.25 inches)

January 18, 2015

Avery "grew" 2 ¼ inches during her surgery. Before (left) and after (right). Photos and graphic by Andrew Butters.

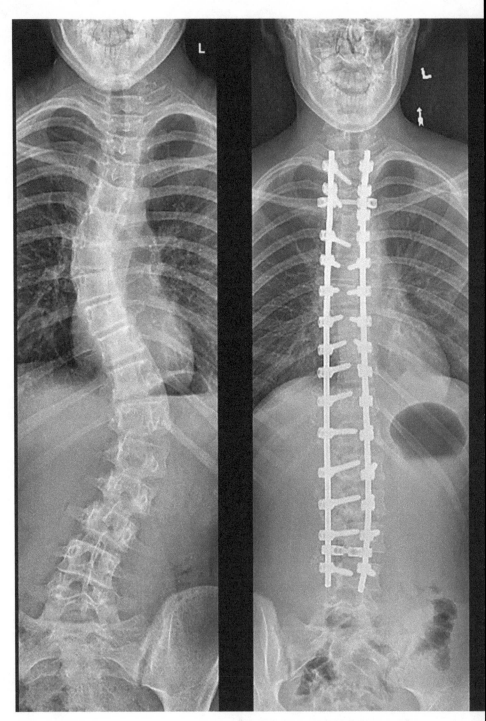

Before and after x-rays taken from the front and side. (Personal Medical Record)

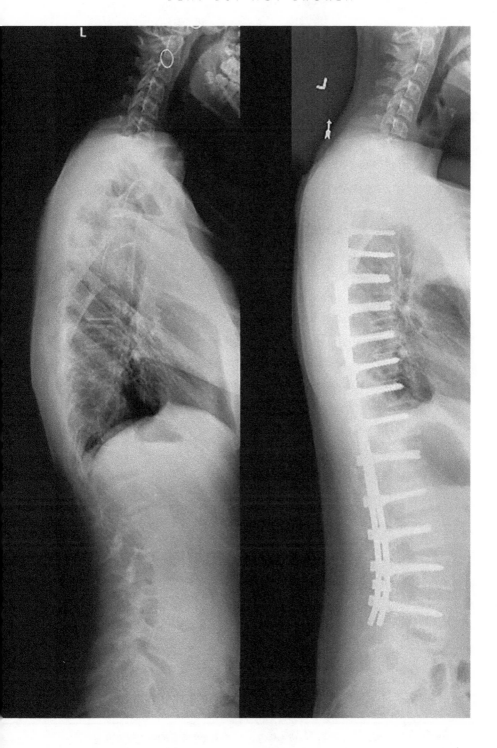

ANDREW: A PICTURE AND A SONG
January 30, 2015 (Post Op Day 10, 2 Days Home)

Today we travelled back down to McMaster Children's Hospital to visit Dr. Missiuna at his fracture clinic for our first post-discharge appointment. As with most visits to the hospital we spent more time finding parking and waiting than we do anything else. It's not normally a big deal but Pants was experiencing the worst pain she says she's felt since she came out of surgery. I suspect her latest dose of pain meds hadn't kicked in yet and the 45 minute journey in the car couldn't have been comfortable. At any rate, they got us into a room so she could lie down and she started to feel better.

Doctor Missiuna came in eventually and took the bandage off her back that was covering up her stitches. He said the wound looked great and that she should take a shower! He also said that she'd start to feel a lot better after about three weeks post-surgery and that part-time school could occur then, with a gradual approach to returning to full-time school as her pain and fatigue levels allow.

We asked about physio and he said that would start at about three months post op. We asked about her body movement and how long it would be before she started to move around more naturally and get used to her new body. He said that at six to twelve weeks they start to feel more comfortable, and that she's still ahead of the curve.

Then, he showed us what we've been eager to see since she got out of surgery. The latest set of x-rays! I asked for a CD of the x-rays from the hospital and they (reluctantly) agreed so I've taken the liberty of including a side-by-side before-and-after view for your enjoyment. Again, I couldn't get the scaling quite right but you get the idea. All I can say is, holy smokes, that's a lot of hardware.

The two images on the left pretty much say it all. She's going to have to get used to having so much of her spine rigid, but look at it! That's one good-looking posture. No more deformation. No more risk of damage to her lungs or other internal organs.

On the way home we stopped to get some Subway and left Pants in the car. As I left she said, "Don't take too long. I'm probably worth a lot of money with all this metal in me." I love that she's still got her sense of humour.

Before this all went down I was talking to my friend and former band mate Jim. I asked him if he thought he could write a song for Pants. She absolutely loves music, and Jim's such a compassionate person (and a talented musician to boot), I figured this was a great idea. Well, today Jim and his band Woot Suit Riot released a song that I can only describe as amazing. Watching the video brought a tear to my eye and as soon as Pants wakes up from her nap I'm going to show it to her. She's heard a rough cut that was missing the harmonies but she was high as a kite at the time so it'll be nice for her to listen to it and see the video with her head less cloudy.

Thank you, Jim and Woot Suit Riot, for doing this. It's an absolutely wonderful gesture and an absolutely wonderful song for an absolutely wonderful girl who we are absolutely proud to call our daughter.

https://youtu.be/vvBehuraQ84

—Dad

JODI: JUST A FEW RANDOM THOUGHTS
January 31, 2015 (Post Op Day 11, 3 Days Home)

Avery, as a twelve-year old girl, does not own many button-up tops. Button-up tops, however, are the only kind she can get on. Those, and spaghetti-strap tank tops that she can step in to and pull up. She is still finding herself warm most often, so the tank tops work in the house, and I bought her a new button-up to go with one she got at Christmas for when we need to go out. She is gaining strength and flexibility every day, so think she will be back in sweaters shortly, but if not, we may need a new wardrobe to account for her added height anyway.

I don't recall if we mentioned how her hips, knees and ankles were all cut up from the rigors of surgery, so she is also finding that only a few of her underpants are comfortable as most of them the band runs right across her scabby hip bone.

Today we left her home for a few hours with one of her friends—she doesn't need constant care but I also am not ready to leave her home alone. On day one she could not put the feet up on the La-Z-Boy, but now she can—

but she also can still get stuck leaning too far back and cannot pull herself up enough to get out of the chair, so someone to rescue her is a good idea.

I told her my signal to start talking about school again is when I see her reading, so she tried today, but couldn't keep her focus to make it through a chapter. She is still on the good drugs, so I give it another week before she starts thinking properly again. She is also curious how she will handle sitting in her desks, as she can currently only handle being up at the table for about fifteen minutes before she needs to recline or full on lie down.

She is still using the jerry-rigged safety rail to get in and out of bed—I knew we were keeping that old sewing chair for a reason! But she pretty much skips down the stairs, so that came back like nothing.

Yesterday I was on a quest for a bath bench, which I found, but then had a laugh in the evening after Andrew went to install it—I seriously forgot the kids have a one-piece bath/shower thing, so there is no lip on the wall side for the bench to rest on—Andrew made it work, though, and Avery enjoyed her first shower in ten days.

She has had to lose her modesty, as there have been a number of things she never would have done in my presence before surgery that have happened post-surgery. Yesterday she called me (on the walkie-talkies—it is so convenient to have these as we are past baby monitors in this house) to come help her dry off after the shower as she still can't balance and bend with any ease. But she was able to get her arms up high enough to brush her hair, so still progress.

Otherwise, as long as we have pain meds, a pillow and some water she can handle most anything we have thrown at her. She eats dinner at the table with us, but gets exhausted by the effort to cut up her food. Her first food requests were all finger foods, I thought for ease of eating, but she later told me that our utensils weigh too much—things I have never considered before.

Before her appointment in Hamilton yesterday she asked if we could go out somewhere. By mid-appointment she had fully changed her mind. I am hoping she will be up for a visit to school this week—her classmates have been amazing and I think it will do her soul good to see a few more of them in person.

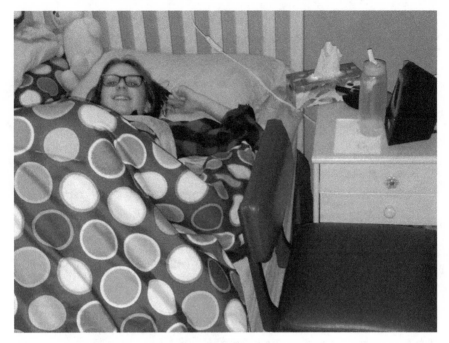

Sewing chair guard rail in Avery's bedroom. (Family Photo)

That's all. Just a few random things in case anyone is reading this as a guidance document for their own kid.

—Mom

AVERY: PANTS WRITES!

February 3, 2015 (Two Weeks Post Op, 6 Days Home)

Hi! Nice to talk to all you guys again. I'm healing up quite nicely and I'm sorry that I haven't posted in a while, I've been a bit distracted with everything else but I'm going to post about all that right now.

The first thing I remember after coming out of surgery is my parents saying it was nine o'clock. The next thing I remember is getting a Popsicle because I burped which I felt stupid but apparently is actually really important. The next thing after that that I remember is standing up and walking to the washroom. That also seemed to be quite special to everyone else and I understand because that one was also a big deal to me. Right then I could feel how difficult it was

125

going to be to do everything else I had to do, like walk upstairs, sit upright for long periods of time and get out of bed without handles to help. It was right then that I really realized how drastic what they had done to me was. For goodness sake, I have 27 screws and two metal rods in my body and they expect me to be able to touch my toes, put on socks and shoes, and live like a normal person. I was terrified, but at the same time I was amazed at how much I could already do. I could already get up. I could walk a little bit and I could go to the washroom. That all may seem really small and insignificant to you guys but it all seems so big at the moment. It all seems so important.

I hope you can learn from my words, and I hope that you never have to do what I had to do.

Thanks for reading.

—Princess Pants

JODI: 17 DAYS POST-OP
February 6, 2015 (Post Op Day 17, 9 Days Home)

So here we are at the end of week 3—seriously? Three weeks? Well no, seventeen days, but the end of three weeks that I have not been at work and the bulk of this adventure began. Avery's aunt was by yesterday and couldn't get over the difference from her hospital visit two weeks ago and now. And how tall Avery is! This twelve-year-old towers over her aunt, and that made Avery smile.

Since Avery clearly does not need constant attention, I have been taking advantage of the time and exercising a little in the basement. Well, today Avery came down to hang out. Since I was at the balance game portion of my Wii fit activities, Avery thought she might like to try as well. So she managed to do six minutes of activities, including deep breathing, basic step (which was funny to watch as she isn't so coordinated) and the soccer ball head butt one. But then she needed to rest. I still think six minutes is better than no minutes, and she was very pleased with herself for having accomplished even that.

In other news, she is almost fully off the meds—she took one at bedtime last night, but hasn't had anything since. We'll see if she feels she needs the night-time one tonight, but I think she could manage on Tylenol—how crazy is that?!? This kid's ability to heal astounds me.

One common theme we have no-ticed is that if she over-exerts herself, she gets an upset tummy later in the day—but she is also quicker at excusing herself to lie down as needed.

So now that the mind-fogging meds are leaving her system, I will contin-ue to watch for those signs of readiness to start heading back to school—my avid reader has not picked up a book in weeks—mind you she also just started watching Grey's Anatomy on Netflix, so I may have lost her for a few more weeks (she did wonder if these people all just signed consent forms so they could film them in the hospital and I explained they were all actors—then she mentioned how good those surgeons seem—had to explain that they are also actors...). She tries to sit up a little each day, but still prefers to be mostly, if not fully, reclined; but I think that will come along soon, too.

—Mom

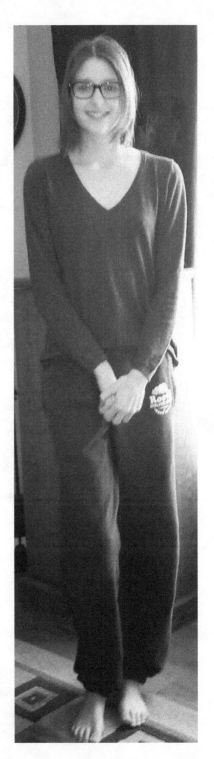

Avery, seventeen days after surgery.
(Family Photo)

JODI: THREE WEEKS POST SURGERY

February 11, 2015 (Post Op Day 22, Two Weeks Home) and All Is Well

We have hit the three-week post-surgery mark, and of course Pants continues to amaze us. While I keep waiting for the moment when she picks up a proper book to read, she has made advancements in her ability to concentrate and reason—through playing Paper Mario on the Wii in the basement or Zelda on the Wii U upstairs. Both require reading and some logic to advance through, so I take it as a win.

And her appetite is back—though she needs to eat smaller meals at several points through the day—but I have read that is better for the body anyway.

Oh, and she is off the heavy pain meds altogether—we have kept a small supply, but I think they will be disposed of before long. She can take Tylenol or Advil as she needs, which she asked for today—though not for her back, but rather her legs—she thinks she might be having a growth spurt!

She can shower mostly standing, but likes to have the bench available, if just to enjoy the warm water running over her back. I was helping to dry her hair and noted that the top two Steri-Strips have curled up at both sides, so I went to remove them and she panicked and screamed not to take them off—seems she is a little concerned she will rip right open without them. So I left them and reassured her that that is not at all the case.

We are off for a pedicure—fingers crossed this isn't too much for her, then after a rest and some dinner she is going to stop by to say hi to Yoga Mike and the class she practiced with. I am so very thankful she and Andrew attended this class together—the number of times people remarked at her leg strength while in the hospital was always responded to with a mention of squats and yoga practice—and every single person who heard this paused for a moment to think about it then nodded as if to acknowledge it made sense. A few even asked her a little more about it. Hopefully in a few months she can start back again.

Today we researched bus routes and schedules as an option to get her home from school—though I will also check with a local taxi company to see what we can do—I don't foresee her walking the two kilometres home from school again this school year, but who knows—maybe once the snow *clears she will enjoy a two-kilometre walk with her brother. The bus runs every thirty minutes from right outside her school, and in under fifteen minutes has her 200 meters from home—we may take a test run this week to see how it goes as I don't think she has ever rode a city bus in her life, and definitely not alone.*

We almost made it out for a pedicure, but then she started to cry. Maybe it was too much. She said she wanted to go, she showered and got dressed—we even had her shoes on. Another day. She just needed a rest. I think she is so terribly freaked out about not being able to control how she is feeling or the fear that she will start hurting and not be able to do anything about it—she honestly was looking like she was when we were last at Dr. Missiuna's and she desperately needed to lie down. So she is lying down. Hopefully the trip to the yoga studio will be a success tonight.

And just as I was leaving to pick up the Dude from school, Avery's teacher called to see how she was doing—I heard 'awesome' then had to leave. Since I am driving anyway, I normally drive home one of Avery's friends—and today she asked if she could come for a visit. I think this day has come together just fine.

—Mom

AVERY: I'M GOING TO SCHOOL!
February 16, 2015 (Post Op Day 27, 19 Days Home)

Hi there. I'm back and I'm here to tell you about all the exciting adventures I've had since we last talked. First we try to go to the pedicure place but I got a little bit scared so we ended up not going, then the next day I went to visit my school. It was really fun getting to see everyone! The teacher even brought donuts! A couple hours after that we went to the pedicure place and got our nails done, but they took a little longer than we thought they would, so we were a little late picking my brother up from school. Two days after that I went to visit my mom's work for a baby shower and pizza. That was also really cool. I sat up for about half an hour, but then I had to take a walk. After the walk I realized that I really needed to lie down, so we left to go home. But what I really wanted to talk about was tomorrow. Tomorrow I get to go to school. I mean actually go to school, not full time but just for a little bit. We're hoping for an hour but we might only get half an hour or so. Still it's really exciting! Have a nice day!

—Princess Pants

JODI: THE GREAT RETURN
February 17, 2015 (Post Op Day 28, 20 Days Home)

Avery's first day back at school lasted about thirty minutes. I decided I would just wait outside the school in my car so we could make a quick return home. It also became quite apparent that a taxi will be the better option—at least until she gets up to half days, at which point we will consider revisiting the bus as an option. She stayed in bed for nearly three hours when we returned home. We'll see how that plays out again tomorrow. :)

And tonight she came running down the stairs visibly vibrating and unable to speak—turns out she pulled off a couple of the Steri-Strips and was rather concerned she would split in two. We reassured her that the strips are in fact supposed to come off and perhaps should be coming off, and she settled down and went back up to bed.

That's all for tonight.

—Mom

ANDREW: A NEW ROUTINE
February 18, 2015 (Post Op Day 29, Three Weeks Home)

It's been a while since I posted so I thought I'd chime in with a few observations and thoughts.

I've been back at work on a normal schedule for more than two weeks. I get up early, being careful to not wake Jodi up on my way out of the bedroom. 50% success rate so far! I get to work before 7:30 am and stick around until 4:15 pm or 4:30 pm. By the time I get home Jodi has made some fantastic dinner and even done some of the dishes. (Best. Wife. Ever.)

Throughout the day I get text messages of Pants's progress and I have to tell you, it's always the highlight of my day.

Pants is walking better, and moving around in general much more naturally every day. We're told it is going to be six to twelve weeks before she starts to feel "normal" again so to see visible progress in that direction every day is just great. We're looking into taxis for her to get home from school until she's comfortable enough to walk from the bus stop to our house which likely won't be until after the snow clears.

Our superstar patient did a full hour at school today! That is such a big step and bodes well for getting her back reading again. Jodi sent me a picture of the part of her back where the Steri-Strips finally fell off and the scar looks good. Nice clean cut, not too wide. Every day I find a new reason to be impressed with the care she's received and with her in general.

Sorry, this post is all over the place.

Things I've noticed:

• I'm still walking around with this tension in my upper body. It's not near as bad as the first week after surgery but it's still there. I'm told this could take a while to subside.

• I am still sleeping like crap most nights. As an insomniac who was sleeping not-too-badly before the surgery, this is frustrating. Some nights are not too bad though and that gives me hope.

• Pants does at least two things every day that make me so proud.

• I'm really going to miss having Jodi home all day. If she's even half as productive in her office they're going to love having her back.

• The Dude is handling everything quite well, but I have noticed he's more cuddly and asking for more hugs, two things I am more than happy to provide in great excess.

• *I never get tired of showing people the before and after x-ray pictures and before and after height picture.*

The next phase starts when Jodi goes back to work. I think she'll drive the kids into school and then Avery will take a cab home whenever she feels she's had enough, eventually working her way toward a full day, after which I'll tweak my work schedule to pick her up or she'll take the bus so she only has to walk the last couple hundred meters.

—Dad

JODI: WE HAVE READING!
February 22, 2015 (Post Op Day 33, 25 Days Home)

Last night when I went up to bed around 10:30 I noticed Avery's bedroom was still lit up—assuming she had fallen asleep with the lights on, I went in—but no, she was still awake READING! It has been a month since she has

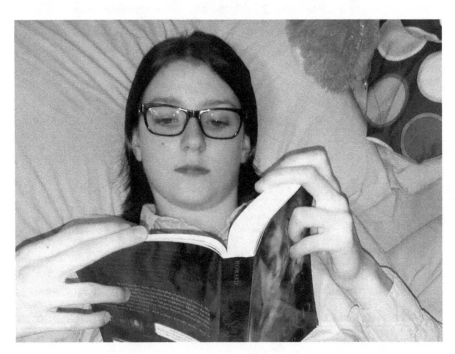

It took a month, but she finally picked up a book. (Family Photo)

had the focus to read anything, so this is a moment we have been waiting for. Shout out to her teacher for the gift of books as that was what she finally found interesting enough to pick and keep reading I am sure by now that book is done.

Avery has been complaining of sore legs this week, and my non-medical assessment is that she really needs some better arch support as her knees are pronating—so for now she is wearing her croc slip on sandals and we will see about something a little better—Birkenstocks or Mephistos, but we need it to get a little nicer out first I think.

—Mom

JODI: ORTHOPEDIC SHOES AND A SCAR
February 27, 2015 (Post Op Day 38, 30 Days Home)

Avery is healing up nicely. She has been to school every day this week and says she has been participating. She is all set up to take a taxi home from school starting next week once I return to work (has it been six weeks

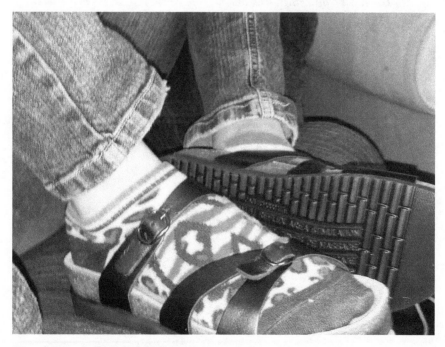

New footwear. (Family Photo)

already?!?) We are hoping to get her to 1.5 hours at school next week, but she will let us know what she needs.

This week's excitement involved the purchase of some fancy orthopaedic sandals for Avery to wear around the house to help address her pronating knee.

Otherwise, her scar is healing up nicely and the Steri-Strips are slowly but surely coming off.

Look at that cute little waist!

I am pleased to say that that is really all I have to report. Things are progressing well and Avery remains ever positive.

—Mom

JODI: MAKE THAT A BAD-ASS SCAR
March 1, 2015 (Post Op Day 38, 30 Days Home)

All the Steri-Strips have been peeled off, and this is the end result, one bad-ass scar!

The scar is a little sticky still, and perhaps a little misleading as her spine in almost perfectly straight but the scar is curved. I suppose the surgeon could only guess as to where her spine would end up once he was done.

Facebook has been super awesome. We will be sure to share all the comments about just how bad-ass she really is.

—Mom

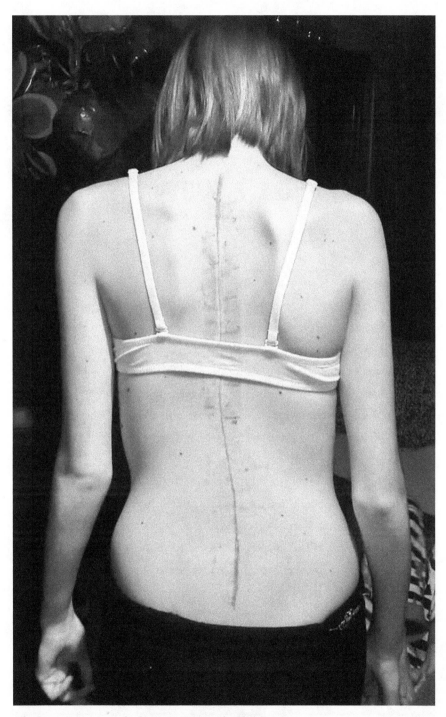

That's one impressive looking scar! (Family Photo)

ELEVEN

HOUSTON, WE HAVE PROGRESS

After the first month of post-surgery, things slowed down quite a bit. One thing I was keeping an eye on was Avery's stamina. Half an hour to Avery's school day was being added every week and at two months after she went under the knife she was managing two hours of class time first thing in the morning. Jodi drove her and The Dude to school and, because she had to go back to work after her six-week leave, had set up an account with a local taxi company so that Avery could call for a cab when she felt tired and come home without having to worry about having any money on her.

Remember how I mentioned that the hard part was going to be slowing her down? It was one hundred percent true. Between March and June Avery's progress was nothing short of spectacular. On Avery's seventy-fourth day after returning home from the hospital she went for a short bike ride. One day, Avery managed to spend more than four hours at school and then attend a fundraiser for Canadian Blood Services that I was holding in my office later in the afternoon.

Even though we did get quite a bit of cash raised, the fundraiser wasn't designed to raise funds. It was designed to drum up donors for a blood drive. Having donated once previously and once for Avery it was imperative for me to ensure that at least as much as Avery used was properly returned to the blood bank. According to Canadian Blood Services that was somewhere around fifteen donors. Without giving away the details I am happy to report that the goal was met and the event was a complete success.

Due to the fact that the recovery time for this surgery takes close to a year and Avery's surgery was in January, it was guaranteed that she would experience every typical annual event and milestone of a normal year, plus many more that she would celebrate the anniversaries of in the years that followed. Regardless of the event, whether it was a birthday, anniversary, the Day To End Bullying (Pink Shirt Day), the Terry Fox Run, swimming in the lake, riding her bike… Everything became The First Time [Whatever It Was] Since Surgery. These milestone events included one that Jodi and I found quite emotional. McHappy Day.

On a day in early May, McDonalds donates one dollar from Happy Meals (every other day they donate ten cents), Big Mac, and hot McCafé Beverage to Ronald McDonald House charities. Having seen firsthand what that charity provided and having been the recipient of some of their kindness Jodi and I both felt compelled to buy a ton of McDonalds that day. I bought two Happy Meals myself and took all the cash I had on me and in the car at the time and threw it in the drive-through donation bin on my way at the payment window. In fact, I still do that every time I'm at one of their drive-through windows.

JODI: 2 MONTHS POST-SURGERY
March 21, 2015 (52 Days Home)

I had to just look twice at that—has it really only been two months? So much has happened, but of late the happenings are often both so frequent and seemingly minute that I guess none of us stopped to write them down. So here is my list, if I have missed anything else exciting, I am sure Pants or Andrew can do a catch up post.

Avery has mastered getting her taxi, and she books it before we leave in the morning, so we know how long she intends to stay (two hours a day before March break).

On March 13 she had an appointment with her surgeon. He was so pleased with the results he called in another orthopaedic intern or resident to admire his handiwork, and he sent Pants home with screen prints of the before and after so she could show her friends (Andrew and I both keep that as our screen savers on our laptops both home and work).

I learned that the surgeons did not make any lateral bends in her rods, which is to say she is pretty much perfectly straight. All the reading I did beforehand suggested we would be lucky to get her below a 20° curve post-surgery.

Pants learned how awful overdoing it in a day can feel. Following the doctor's appointment (including the 1.5 hours in the car) she wanted to go to school for the afternoon—it was the day before the break and they were going to be watching a movie and a basketball game, so we said fine. I picked her up at 3:00, and she went right up to lie down. Friday was also Andrew's birthday, and that means dinner out. Andrew kindly chose Mandarin Buffet as we knew it could be faster than table service, and we headed out before 5:00. Dinner was yummy, but by 6:30 it was pretty clear Pants was ready to fall over, so we headed home. And at 3:30 am she was up feeling so nauseous and scared of what throwing up was going to do to her back. I got a Gravol in her, but half an hour later she couldn't hold it in—and in her practical way, said well, I threw up in the sink so I didn't have to bend over and it was fine.

She was cleared for floating. Monday night Pants and Andrew went to the Y. Pants wore a scar-baring tankini top—I love that she is so comfortable in her skin (because really, it is a pretty cool scar!)

Pants was excited the other day because she sat up in bed. I didn't get it, until she demonstrated that up until that point she had been rolling to her side and pushing herself up to sitting, but last week she just went right up to sitting. She was quite pleased with this feat.

Her grandmother came for a visit on Thursday and took her in to Waterloo for lunch with Andrew. Her appetite is definitely coming back as she ordered the dinner steak and wedges and got through half of it—then ate the rest for lunch the following day.

Her grandmother brought her a couple of vitamin E treatment to help the scar heal, but Avery has asked if she has to use them, because as I said above, it is a pretty cool scar. We will keep them on hand should she change her mind.

She went out for another float—this time we confirmed she could in fact swim lightly, and that made it even better. I think we will try to get her in the water a little more often.

She walked over to her friend's house to see if she could come over—it isn't far, but it was the longest walk she has done since the surgery. It is so much nicer now that the snow has started to melt.

Yesterday she went to a movie. Another milestone as far as being able to be out and seated in one place for almost two hours, but she also needed a long rest when she got home.

So it is back to school on Monday. As odd as it seems, the new goal is for her to make it to the end of first nutrition break—we are suggesting she use the outdoor time indoors doing some homework. The goal is increased stamina and that break happens every day, so she needs to be able to make it through it before we can add another class into her day.

So there—three weeks of progress, and more happening every day. :)

— Mom

JODI: OUT FOR A RIDE

April 12, 2015 (74 Days Home)

Again it seems like nothing of major concern has happened since the last update, but today it was finally a nice day, and Andrew cleared out of the garage and brought all the bikes down—and Avery just couldn't resist so she went out for a little bike ride! I stood in the driveway the whole time, eagerly wanting to see her come around the corner on her bike. Her brother zoomed down the street and a few moments later, there was Avery—sporting the best posture ever and a smile that could have generated light. Quite honestly, it brought a tear to my eye.

She is up to over four hours a day of school, and adding a little more every week. Really, her recovery is going as good if not better than expected. I think Andrew noted a month ago that the hard part is going to be slowing her down.

She was a little upset last week as we had our first thunderstorms of the season—she texts us every day to say she got home from school ok. Thursday's

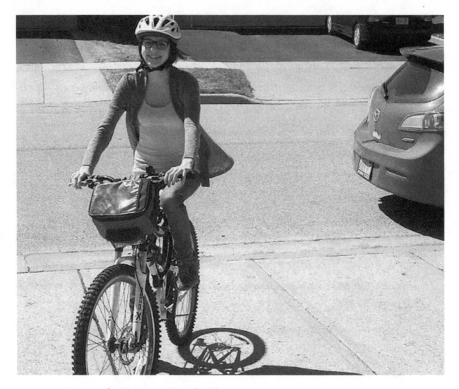

Princess Pants rides again.. (Family Photo)

text included a note about how she was afraid she was at risk for lightning strike due to her new hardware....

And I suppose we passed another milestone—Andrew and I went out in the evening and didn't have a second thought about leaving Avery with her brother. Last month he (ha—both Andrew and AJ) would not have been okay with that as she was still getting too tired and needed to rest, but no one blinked an eye at it last night. Oh how wonderful life is these days.

—Mom

JODI: THE ONE WHERE GOING TO MCDONALD'S MAKES ME CRY

May 6, 2015 (98 Days Home)

Today is McHappy Day and we will be going. It is possible I will make *multiple visits. On any normal day, this is not anything I would do—we maybe have McDonald's a half-dozen times a year, normally on the road or otherwise in a pinch. But today we are going for McHappy Day, and that means the money will be going to support the most wonderful, amazing, kind services of the Ronald McDonald Houses (RMH) and other children's charities.*

I don't know how much we discussed RMH in relation to Avery's surgery, but there is one just across from McMaster. We were provided an application form, I even filled it out—but the idea that we might take a room from a family who was dealing with something worse than back surgery (major back surgery, but we knew she would be coming home once she was able) made me feel bad. Plus, we were something like 2.4 km over the minimum distance—and Dude was going to be home. The RMH room was a godsend, and I for one will do something as trivial as buy a Big Mac—maybe twice—to help make sure that room and the RMH are forever available for people who need them. I really hope you never need them.

And one other little plug—whatever politics you may feel about blood donation—the blood bank always needs your help. You know Avery needed fifteen donors' worth of blood. You might have a friend who has had cancer treatments and needed blood. If you can, please donate. My Princess needed it to safely make it out of surgery—if you could help another parent say the same thing, wouldn't you want to?

—Mom

ANDREW: BENT BUT NOT BROKEN
BLOOD DRIVE UPDATE

May 8, 2015 (100 Days Home!)

As Jodi mentioned in her last post we're having a blood drive in an effort to give back some of what Avery needed to get her through the surgery. Sign-ups have been slowly trickling in, but we're still a few people shy of getting our target number of fifteen donors.

My company, Agfa HealthCare, has one of these old-timey-looking pop-corn machines that they let employees use every Friday. The company buys the popcorn, all you have to do is set up shop and pop the stuff (and clean up everything after) and you can sell popcorn for $2 a bag. The only conditions are:

• You can only send one email to the office promoting your event and one email afterward thanking everyone (so as to not spam / pester everyone).

• The money has to go to a registered charity.

So, in an effort to drum up donors and donations we held a Popcorn Friday in support of Canadian Blood Services today and Princess Pants and The Dude came to work with me this afternoon to help sell popcorn.

My introduction email explained a bit about Avery and how she needed so much blood for her surgery and that we were looking for six more donors to round out our list or cash from popcorn sales to donate to Canadian Blood Services.

Last night, Jodi got this awesome idea to make up t-shirts with pictures of Avery's x-rays on them promoting the blood drive. The kids wore theirs to school and I wore mine to work. They looked awesome and they were a big hit!

I took the kids out of school around 1:00 and brought them into work and we started popping popcorn a little before 2:00. Someone had already given me a $20 donation because they were out of the office for the afternoon so we were off to a great start. Once the smell of the popcorn started wafting through the office it didn't take long for the donations to start rolling in.

By 3:00 we had sold a lot of popcorn and a co-worker suggested that we take some upstairs on the rolling table and see if the office on the third floor wanted any (he tipped us off that they were always in the mood for popcorn).

So we trekked upstairs with eleven bags of popcorn and visited Watsec Cyber Risk Management. Less than ten minutes later we only had one bag left!

We sold a few more before the day came to a close for us (around 4:00) and the final tally was nothing short of amazing:

• $238 ($245) if you include the 5€ note someone gave us.

• Two blood donors for the drive on May 14.

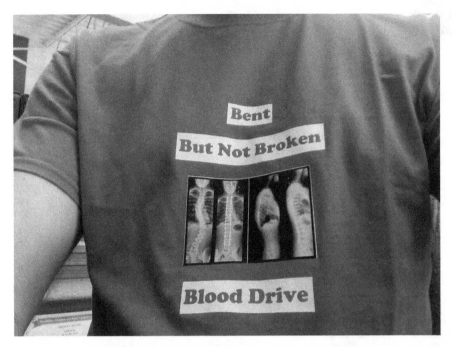

Designer blood drive t-shirts. (Family Photo)

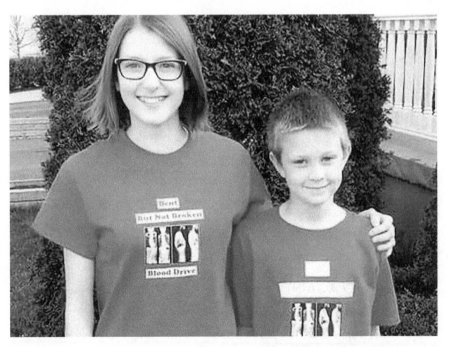

Pants and Dude ready for the blood drive at Andrew's office. (Family Photo)

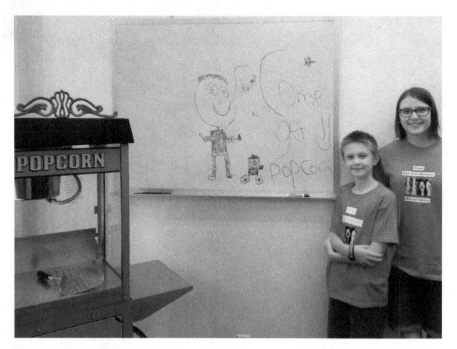

Pants and Dude ready for the blood drive at Andrew's office. (Family Photo)

• One blood donor who can't make the 14th but will donate at another point in the week.

• I even had people tell me they would be away on Friday but would bring in donations on Monday!

All in all, it was an amazing success. The generosity of Agfa HealthCare Waterloo and Watsec Cyber Risk Management is quite something. I am very fortunate to be a part of such a wonderful and caring community.

—Dad

AVERY: HELLO AGAIN

May 15, 2015 (107 Days Home)

Once again, hello, everyone. Yesterday the one thing I failed to mention was that all of this couldn't have happened without the help of my dad. He *planned it, he set in action, and he went through with it. He's the one who has all of the friends who donate blood. Anyways, stuff about my everyday life. I now go to school until 2:30, just half an hour away from a full day. I went to a movie without any adults for the first time ever, and I'm just doing amazing overall. I hope you're all doing as well as me, talk again soon.*

—Princess Pants

TWELVE

HOUSTON, WE HAVE A TEENAGER

If the first few months of healing were any indication I was sure that there was going to be several more emotional moments ahead and I was not disappointed. You see, Avery was set to become a teenage girl and I was not prepared. Oh, I had heard stories about these times from many different sources but had yet to experience it. Up until that point Avery was completely consumed with the lead-up to surgery and the surgery itself, so there was nothing "normal" about it. None of the prognostications I received had come true because none of the prognostications took into consideration the uniqueness of Avery's situation.

So it was easy for me to determine how Avery was doing because all I had to do was look for normal teenager behaviour and I'd know everything was as it should be. If anyone is counting that day came almost exactly five months after surgery—four days after Avery's thirteenth birthday.

Of course, Avery being Avery, the big teenage angst phase lasted all of a couple weeks.

One of the things that Jodi and I noticed over the course of this journey is that Avery didn't complain. She had a couple moments of fear and doubt and expressed her opinions on the matter, but Avery, in her daily interactions with Jodi and I, never complained. Not once. No one would have given it a second thought if she had, but she didn't, even after *The Fall*.

Ah, The Fall.

The Fall was one of those horrible moments where you feel like the worst parent ever and resent your job for making you work when clearly there are more important things going on.

First, a little backstory. Jodi and I have a system for emergencies. If one of us calls the other and it goes to voice mail, if it's an emergency, call right back. This way, if we are otherwise occupied at work we know if we should interrupt what we're doing to answer the phone. Back in June of 2015 it would have been a good idea to have explained this to Avery.

Avery was home alone, as she often was during the times after school and before I got home from work. One day in early June Avery hopped off the couch a little too quickly, got dizzy, and passed out. She awoke on the floor disoriented and in terrible pain. She called me but I was on a work call at the time. I saw her call come through but let it go to voice mail and waited.

No second call.

It didn't occur to me that I had never explained the system to Avery. A short time later Jodi called me. Something was definitely up. Fortunately, I was at my desk. My headset was on and some co-workers from Rhode Island were on a web-based meeting and conference call. I told them something was happening with my wife or daughter and put them on hold while I looked at my phone.

There was one of those floating chat heads from Facebook on my screen. It was Avery's former caregiver, Stephanie. She sent Jodi and I a message telling us that Avery fell. Jodi replied with, "On my way," and Stephanie replied that she was okay but shaken up. I almost lost my lunch but composed myself and checked my voice mail. The message was incoherent hysterics.

Part of me was glad that I knew she was not in any immediate danger because had I answered that call and heard the screaming on the other end I'm not sure how I would have reacted. As it was, I felt relieved that she was in good hands. I called Jodi and told her I was coming home too. I got back to my conference call and gave them a two sentence summary about what happened and ended the call. I told my boss what happened, packed up my stuff, and booted home.

Avery said she felt okay when I got home and she had a scrape from where her back slid down the counter top (how she got turned around in that direction we still don't know). Even though she felt fine, I still called Avery's surgeon to see if she should come in. Avery was due to see him in ten days but we hadn't planned on her falling down. A big concern for us was the fact that we were driving down to Virginia as a family to see Jodi's cousin get married in a couple days. There was no way we were missing that wedding so now it was a matter of if Jodi and Avery would fly or if we'd still all go in the car.

Since Avery was already scheduled to see Dr. Missiuna the following week, he said that we should bring her in just in case. So, in she went, and out she came without any fanfare. According to Dr. Missiuna, Avery's x-rays looked spectacular and she was cleared for the big car trip down to Virginia. Coincidentally, the car ride would end up being about the same length as Avery's surgery was. This gave Avery a bit of perspective on the whole event because she didn't have a clue about very much from the time she went under to the time they took her off the morphine pump.

Summer came and went without any fanfare as well, unless you count a few more healing milestones for Avery (which I certainly do). Dr. Missiuna told Jodi and I that he was taking a cautious approach to Avery's recovery. I neglected to ask Dr. Missiuna how many surgeries he had performed before Avery but I did know that he had a perfect track record. Other surgeons in the United States were touting a six-month return to full activity but the NHS in United Kingdom and our province of Ontario here in Canada recommended at least a one-year gradual return.

By the time summer rolled around Avery was doing some light swimming, lots of walking, and she was back to her old self, reading about one novel per day. Most importantly for me was the fact that Avery's personality was returning to her pre-surgery state. That being a kind and carefree girl who took good care of her little brother when Jodi and I had to work.

Summer was also the time when I was brought to tears by an Australian singer by the name of Vance Joy. That was the time I realized that you truly can find good people everywhere you look.

AVERY: THE FALL

June 10, 2015 (133 Days Home)

Yesterday at 1:30 in the afternoon I went to go get some lunch from the kitchen. I got up off the couch and walked to the kitchen. By the time I got there the head rush from standing up off the couch too quick had caught up to me. I get head rushes when I stand up too fast, and this one was really bad. I passed out, and when I could see again I was lying on the floor in horrible pain. I stood up, slowly, and walked to the phone, all the while crying my eyes out and wailing. I called my dad but got voice mail, so I left a message (as I learned later, all it sounded like was a screaming banshee). So next I called my mom. It rang for a minute, and then just went silent. No buzzing, no mom, no nothing. So I screamed and cried until I remembered that my old babysitter, Stephanie, lived really close, so I called her, and she picked up. I was so relived, that for a brief second, I stopped crying. But only for a second. In my hysterics, I tried to tell her what had happened. You know when you're crying, but trying not to, and you start having these weird jerk pause breaths? Almost like hiccups? That was happening to me. Eventually she got it out of me that I had fallen, and came over right away. By the time she got here I had stopped screaming and was now just crying a lot. She helped me stop crying, and helped me get an ice pack, and then she Facebooked my parents that I had fallen. After a couple minutes my dad called. By then I had stopped crying, mostly, and we had figured out what was hurting. It was just a pinkish line parallel to my scar on my right side (and as we found out later, a bruised tailbone). My mom called minutes later and started to drive home right away. My dad called her and asked when she would be home. Since Stephanie could only stay until 2:30, she said she would be home soon. And she wasn't lying. She was home by not quite two. Stephie stayed a bit longer, but then had to leave. We thanked her immensely. A short while after that my dad got home. He called the doctor and got us an appointment for today. Life went on. I was ok. This morning my mom stayed home and we went to the doctors. We got x-rays and had Subway for lunch, and then we went to the doctor's. The only thing I was nervous about was not being able to go to Virginia for my mom's cousins wedding. Doctor Missiuna said that my x-rays were excellent, that I was fine except *for a contusion (whatever that means), and that I was not allowed to drive to Virginia, but that I could be a passenger. He also cleared me to start physio and yoga. Yes! :) :) when we got back to Cambridge we bought some flowers for Stephie, as that was the least we could do. It was a strange coincidence, as the flower shop lady's stepdaughter had just had the same surgery as me a week ago. That's all I have to say for now. I'll try to update more often.*

Write more later.

—Princess Pants

AVERY: I WAS THINKING LAST NIGHT
June 18, 2015 (141 Days Home)

I want to be a kid again. Shrink me down to six and leave me there. Take me out of this age where I'm responsible for lots of things. Where I'm not little anymore. No longer a child, a kid, where I start preparing for the real world. Where everything I do matters a lot more than it used to. I hate it. I can't stand it. At first I was so excited. It was all I wanted. Now all I want is for it to be over. I wish I could have skipped it. Just gone from child to adult, so I don't have to go through this. Shrink me down to six, before I'm an actual person. At six you're not quite a person yet. You don't have a personality, at least not the one you'll have for the rest of your life. At six even the most outgoing of your class is still a bit shy. At six fart is a word that makes you gasp because someone said a 'bad word'. At six everything mattered in its own way, even if now the things that mattered then seem stupid. At six daddy could pick me up. At six I could sit on mommy's lap. At six cars seemed like a fantastic thing (aside from me getting sick in them). At six life seemed perfect. At six you can have a temper tantrum, go to your room saying you hate your parents, only to come out minutes later crying and saying sorry and that you loved them. At six you got books read to you at night. At six you slept with a night light. At six you knew, with all your heart, no matter what was said and done, that your parents loved you then and will love you forever. Now at times you feel like no one gets you. You want to believe that your parents will always love you but are afraid you will do something wrong. Now everything is scary. I'm afraid

I'll fail school. I'm afraid I'll get fat. I'm afraid I'm too skinny. I'm afraid I'll get hit by a car. I'm afraid I'll get kidnapped. I'm afraid that in high school I'll smoke or take drugs. I'm REALLY scared about that last one. I don't want to be a teenager. I don't want to go to high school. I just want to be a kid again. To not be afraid to go into my parents room if I have a nightmare. To be able to walk around not worrying about what's around the corner. Or about what's ahead of me on life. To be able to snuggle up in my parents arms again. Please let me be a kid again. Please.

—Princess Pants

AVERY: GRADE SEVEN. THE (NOT QUITE) END
June 18, 2015 (141 Days Home)

I wrote this a couple days ago, and forgot to post it, so here it is.

Before I had my surgery was an emotional time for me. I was both terrified and excited. Terrified that I would die in surgery, and excited that if all went well my back would be better forever. On my last day of school my whole class wore tiaras, and one of my teachers got almost all of the seniors to wear ones that they made in class. It made me feel so fantastic. You have no idea how wonderful it felt. We got a picture of my class wearing tiaras, and I've kept it as my background picture on my iPad until just recently. That picture reminds that these people care about me, even just a bit. And I care about them. I've known most of them since grade two, and some since grade five, but I've still know them long enough to be sad that this year is over. Two whole months not seeing some of them. I know that I still get to see them next year, so it's not REALLY the end but it still feels like it. We're not leaving to go to high school, but we've started preparing. I mean, we just survived our first year as seniors, doing different subjects in gym, new stuff at track, millions of new things that we learned in all subjects, our first year of math in English instead of in French (which by the way, makes it a lot easier to understand), our first year with history instead of social studies, our first year starting to get points towards the award of excellence, and much more. This year has been full of good and bad things and I'm happy I got to spend it with people I did. Even the nurses and doctors were pretty nice. Thank you to everyone who's been with me on this journey, even if you didn't follow it as it happened. And I hope everything I've written (and will continue to write) has and will help you in some way as it has me.

Thank you all.

—*Princess Pants*

JODI: DIVING BOARD!
July 26, 2015 (179 Days Home)

*https://www.facebook.com/jodi.wilksbutters/videos/
vb.527281293/10153376674486294/?type=2&theater*

AVERY: JUST A RANDOM WEIRD THOUGHT
July 30, 2015 (183 Days Home)

So. My scar is thicker at the bottom, and I was touching it, and I suddenly realized what it feels like. You know when you get a new book and it has that plastic wrap over it? When you run your hand over that? That's why my scar feels like when I touch it but softer. And instead of there being a book inside of the plastic wrap, it's my spine, and instead of plastic wrap it's fresh new skin.

Just a random, weird thought.

—*Princess Pants*

ANDREW: THE JOY OF VANCE
August 17, 2015 (201 Days Home)

Jodi and I were talking on the way up to the cottage. We both noticed that Princess Pants, not once throughout this whole ordeal, has even so much as mumbled a single complaint. Not one. Zero. She went to hell and back at a time in her life when she should have been looking forward to becoming a teenager and she never complained. Sure, she had moments where she was down, or scared, or wrote something on the blog like "I want to be a kid again," which is perfectly healthy and we're glad she had the outlet to do it, but day-to-day

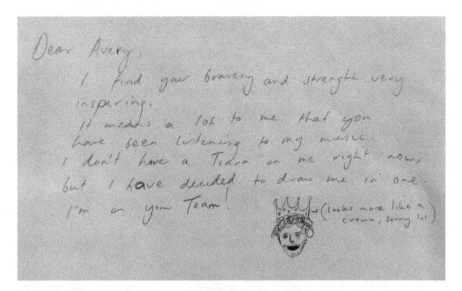

Handwritten letter (while out on tour!) from Vance Joy.

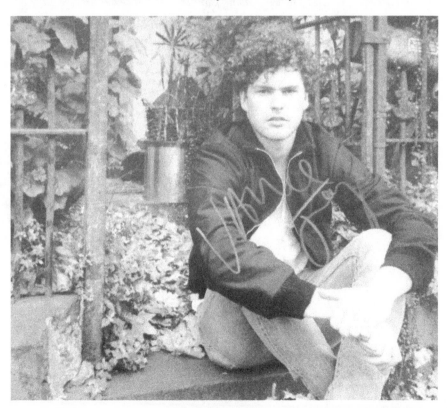

Vance Joy. (Letter and photograph courtesy Vance Joy. Reprinted with permission.)

complaints? Zip. She took the really crappy hand she was dealt and she accepted it, and that makes it even more amazing.

So, on June 27 I did something hoping it would pay off and bring a big ole smile to Princess Pants's face: I sent an email to Taylor Swift and Vance Joy. Taylor is on a world tour and Vance is one of her opening acts and Pants loves them both (more so Vance, I think). I explained in my email what Pants went through and how she listened to their music and told them the story of her class wearing tiaras on her last day of school before surgery. I asked them if they would be so kind as to mention Pants in a tweet or send her an email or autographed picture. Somewhat jokingly I said that if they had a picture of them wearing a tiara that would be positively epic.

Well, on August 6 I got a FedEx envelope from Vance Joy addressed to Pants. It looked like it would hold an 8x10 photo and figured that Vance's manager or PR person sent one along from the stack they have in the office (I'm sure he signs a bunch every time he sees his manager for just such an occasion). Pants was up at the cottage with Grandma that day and we were to bring it up to her the next day.

Jodi noticed that the envelope was mailed overnight delivery and came from Edmonton and mentioned that Vance and Taylor were just in Edmonton. I reckoned at this point that what was in the envelope was probably more than just an 8x10 glossy off the stack in the office. I was right. I decided that I would record Pants opening the envelope to see if her reaction was YouTube worthy.

It was.

https://youtu.be/8uOD_5BaGEg

Inside were an autographed picture and a hand-written note.

Dear Avery,

I find your bravery and strength inspiring. It means a lot to me that you have been listening to my music. I don't have a tiara on me right now, but I have decided to draw me in one. I'm on your team!

(Looks more like a crown, sorry lol)

The video above tells you all you need to know about how well this worked out. Her reaction brought a tear to my eye and still does every time I watch it (which is often).

Thank you, Vance Joy, for making my daughter feel like the happy, elated, giddy teenager she deserves to be.

—Dad

THIRTEEN

BACK TO SCHOOL

One of my main concerns that I never vocalized was how her classmates would respond going into eighth grade. I'm not sure why it was a concern for me, after all, the support that everyone in Avery's school showed her to this point was nothing short of tear-inducing. But eighth grade was a different beast. For Avery it meant that she was among the most senior-ranking students in the school. Kids were no doubt looking forward to high school and started to split off into various factions.

I mentioned earlier, I started to notice this in seventh grade but it wasn't a concern then because Avery was going through her lead-up to surgery and then her surgery and recovery. Everybody loved Avery, and rightly so, because she went through hell and still came out the other side the same Avery—only stronger.

By the start of September, however, all the other kids had myriad opportunities to get together and do loads of summery things. Avery spent a lot of time at home or with Grandma and Grandpa up at the cottage but not a whole lot with her friends. She spent quality time with some of her close pals, for sure, but it was definitely less than it would have been under more normal circumstances.

It turns out that, as usual, I had nothing to worry about. Yes, the kids in school splintered off into their various groups, but based on what I knew about Avery's classmates, the way it unfolded didn't come as a surprise. One of the girls started dating one of the boys and I wondered if this would have any impact on Avery's socializing.

Nope.

Avery was devoted to her friends, especially the ones that showed her the most support throughout her ordeal, and was concerned more with the resumption of normal activities. In fact, as you will read, there weren't many updates to the blog from September to December and they were Avery's, and focused around yoga, gym class, physiotherapy, and intramural sports.

I never considered Avery to be the most athletic person but she was always active and participating in various sports at school or in the evenings. Jodi and I insisted on it. What was obvious, though, was Avery was missing the activity, and with her progress ahead of schedule it was nice to see her so excited about getting her feet moving again.

There was a lot of time between the start of school and December, when Avery saw Dr. Missiuna for her almost-one-year checkup. I have mentioned before how Dr. Missiuna took a cautious approach to healing, telling us that the only real way to know that Avery's spine was healed was to wait it out. For me, the only thing on my mind for those four months was seeing Dr. Missiuna and hearing the words "cleared for all activities."

AVERY: YOGA

September 18, 2015 (233 Days Home)

I went to yoga today. For the first time. In FOREVER. And it was amazing. I had so much fun. It was really nice to see yoga Mike again. I felt so, so, FANTASTIC afterwards. I know this post is short, but I just had to let you know. Write again soon.

—*Princess Pants*

AVERY: HELLO AGAIN

October 28, 2015 (273 Days Home)

So I really should have posted last Wednesday, but I forgot, what with all of the excitement. I got to do gym last Wednesday. It was AWESOME. It felt so good to finally be able to do stuff again. It was actually supposed to be last TUESDAY, but my class didn't have gym on Tuesday, so I didn't get to do it. My teacher was nice enough to let us have QDPA (Qualified Daily Physical Activity) though. But anyways, I hope you're all doing okay, because I've been feeling fantastic. We carved our pumpkins for Halloween last night. Mine is a cat with devil horns and a set of wings. I think it looks pretty awesome if I do say so myself. Happy Halloween everyone, or if you don't celebrate Halloween, have a good rest of the week and weekend. So yeah. Gym. I never realized how much I missed it until I got it back.

I'll try to update more often.

—Princess Pants

AVERY: HELLO AGAIN. AGAIN
October 29, 2015 (274 Days Home)

I know it's only been a day but I already have more exciting news. So we went to the physiotherapists, and Jay got me to do my leg-y stuff, and all I did was two things, when he said that all I need is some stronger bands, and that I don't have to come back unless Dr. Missiuna says so or a problem arises. So, yeah. I no longer have to go to the physiotherapists because I'm just that bendy. Not actually, but still.

Talk to you as soon as something interesting happens.

Happy Halloween Saturday.

—Princess Pants

AVERY: JUST AN UPDATE
November 24, 2015 (300 Days Home!)

So, today was my first time getting to do intramurals, which is an orga-nized tournament of a certain sport that happens during my nutrition breaks at school, and it was really fun. In other not so exciting news, I went to the family doctor last Wednesday, and she said that I seemed to be doing good. And this Wednesday, tomorrow, I get to go with my class to visit HIGH SCHOOL, *which is really scary, and really exciting. Everything is going amazing, I have about fifteen books I have to read, and Christmas is coming up. My brother and I built snowmen on Sunday, which is when I realized I spent ALMOST ALL OF last winter in a bed, and it was awesome to play in the snow in NO-VEMBER, because Canada loves the cold. It also meant I got hot chocolate ^_^*

Have a nice end of November.

—Princess Pants

FOURTEEN

ONE YEAR

Twelve months is a long time to spend worrying but as a parent it seems that that is our most frequent activity. Add to that a child who is going through something traumatic over which you have zero control and worrying becomes all you know. It is all-consuming, it is exhausting, but if you're lucky it is also temporary.

I've said from the beginning of this that of all the stuff that's out in the world that can screw up a child, Avery got lucky. Avery was lucky because she got dealt a hand that could be played. It sure wasn't a pair of aces, but it wasn't a junk hand you give up on either. Avery was fixable, and that's exactly what Dr. Missiuna and all the fine health care professionals and support staff at McMaster Children's Hospital in Hamilton, Ontario did. All it cost Jodi and I was a few dollars and a lot of worrying.

In Avery's case the cost was much greater. This surgery cost her more than a year of her life. At a time when everyone else was concerned with being a kid and becoming a teenager, Avery was concerned with whether or not she would be able to walk again. Avery was concerned with whether or not she would have any friends when she finally returned to "normal". Avery was concerned with whether or not she would look deformed. Avery was concerned with whether or not she would be able to do everything she was able to do before.

At one of Avery's appointments before the surgery Dr. Missiuna told a story about an elite American athlete, a swimmer, who missed qualifying for the Olympics by fractions of a second. This young man underwent the same surgery Dr. Missiuna was to perform on Avery and his point was that when it was all said and done she would have the physical capabilities to do just about anything she wanted.

Now, from May of 2014 to December of 2015 is a long time for a child to be left wondering if Dr. Missiuna's claim was true. That's nineteen months of my child wondering if she would have the opportunity to do any of the things she loved again. So, when Jodi and I took Avery to see Dr. Missiuna for her (almost) one year checkup the only thing on all our minds was whether or not she could go back to being a kid again.

We weren't waiting in the room very long after Avery had her x-rays taken before Dr. Missiuna came in and sat down and spoke the words we had been waiting to hear since this ordeal began.

"Avery is cleared for all activities."

Full-contact sports are out (hockey, football, rugby, and the like), as is trampoline, but everything else is on the table. Volleyball, Avery's favourite, was starting in a few weeks and you can bet your butt she wanted to be signed up for that. And then there was skiing. Before the surgery Avery took ski lessons and was out on the hill every week. Could Avery ski? Yes, but keep off the Black Diamond hills and avoid moguls. With a class field trip to the local ski hill on the horizon the news that Avery was cleared for all activities was music to her ears.

This also meant that Jodi and I could go back to worrying about the same old regular stuff parents worry about. Which was fine by me.

ANDREW: MINUTES

January 9, 2016 (346 Days Home)

I was working in a video store sometime in the mid-1990's and we had The Beatles "Yellow Submarine" on the television for the customers to stare at while they were browsing for a movie to rent. The song "When I'm Sixty-Four" came on and the movie counted out a full minute. That was probably the first moment I was consciously aware of the fact that one minute is actually a very long time.

Watch the clock or your watch for one minute before you keep reading. Sit and do nothing but stare. Continue reading when you're done.

Welcome back. Did a minute feel like a long time or a short time? For me back in 1990-something, it felt like a long time. Regardless of how long it felt to you, I want you to multiply that by six hundred and sixty. Now imagine sitting around for that many rotations of the second hand on your clock or watch. Now, imagine that during this marathon of minutes your daughter was being cut open from neck to tailbone and having chrome/cobalt rods affixed directly to her spine with twenty-seven titanium screws, each one secured in place to part of a vertebra that needed to have a hole drilled in it. Finally, imagine that the margin for error on the location of each hole was only 2 millimeters (funnily enough, that's about 1/64 of an inch on either side of the hole) and that any move outside that margin of error could result in your daughter being paralyzed. Now, does that feel like a long time?

Pants was in surgery for roughly 660 minutes. Six hundred and sixty minutes that felt like an eternity. Since then, so many more minutes have gone by, and to me, it feels like they passed in just a fraction of the time.

At the time of me typing this sentence, it has been 509,192 minutes since Avery got out of surgery and 509,072 minutes since we were allowed to see her. She was lying in a bed hooked up to three IVs and a breathing tube down her throat. Her face was swollen and she had sores and cuts. She had hives all over her body from a reaction to something in surgery (possibly some of the five litres of blood they needed to transfuse). She looked like she had been hit by a truck, and that is the exact analogy the surgeon used when he was talking to us. Imagine your daughter had been hit by a truck and she would not wake up for another 720 minutes. Seven hundred and twenty consecutive loops of the video. Sixty more loops than the eternity of hell you just went through.

That was 508,357 minutes ago, and quite possibly one of the scariest, heart-wrenching, but also the most reassuring minutes of my entire life. My little princess would be okay. The minutes that followed, just about every one of the more than half a million that have passed, have been all good. For me, that's the most amazing part of this whole journey. Pants never complained. Her attitude remained positive the entire way and her recovery followed

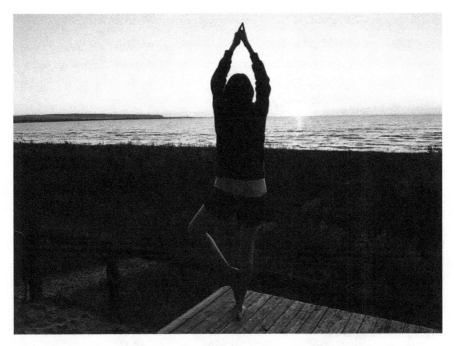

Sunset, tree pose at Wasaga Beach. (Family Photo)

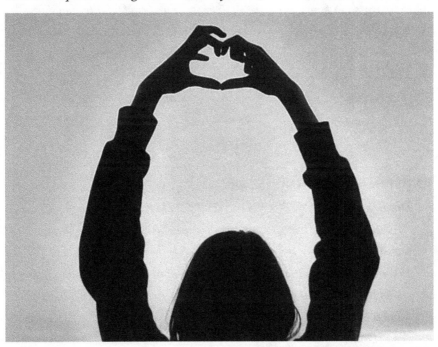

Sunset, with love. (Family Photo)

the same path. About 445,768 minutes ago I wrote that the hard part was going to be slowing her down. With all the talk of kids today being coddled and "soft," all you need to do is find one facing a bit of adversity to see just how wrong that assertion is.

Approximately 15,690 minutes from now I'm going to be away on business. I will be alone and thinking of my little girl. At that moment, it will have been exactly one year, 525,600 minutes since I walked her into surgery, and with tears in both our eyes kissed her on the forehead and watched her fall asleep. Of all the minutes between those two dates on the calendar marking one complete journey around the sun, there were more filled with stress, anxiety, fear, and emotional torture than any family should have to endure. But the good news is that those minutes were but a fraction of the total minutes that have passed since. The really good news is that at 8:01 AM on January 20, 2016, every single one of those minutes will be in the past.

At that time, Princess Pants will be starting a different journey around the sun and our family will have an unknown number of minutes remaining to work with. With any amount of luck, it will be millions upon millions, which would please me greatly, because the last 508,407 seem to have passed a little too quickly.

Hug the ones you love and make every minute count.

—*Dad*

ANDREW: HAPPY ANNIVERSARY

Sunday, January 24, 2016 (One Year + 3 Days Post Surgery)

I was uncertain what the anniversary of Pants's surgery would bring. A year ago I was going through something that, even as a writer, I found almost completely indescribable. Part of me hoped that January 20, 2016, would feel triumphant—a giant middle finger to scoliosis and all the fear, trauma, and anxiety it caused my daughter as well as myself and the rest of our family.

It didn't.

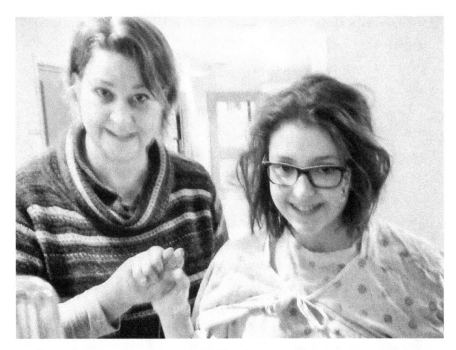

Walking. January 23, 2015. (Family Photo)

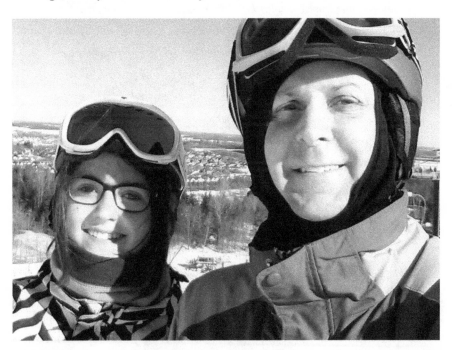

Skiing. January 23, 2016. (Family Photo)

Instead, it was a slightly numbed and not-quite-disassociated repeat of the original emotions. It followed me around all day. Every minute I found to sit and reflect took me back to the same time of day a year ago. It shouldn't have been like that. At least, that's not what my expectation was, and it was all quite a bit more overwhelming than I think I was prepared to manage, especially considering that I was out of the country and couldn't even seek refuge in the warm embrace of Princess Pants, The Dude, or my wife.

Then, yesterday happened.

Yesterday morning I woke up and checked my email and did some Facebooking as I normally do and I took a gander at the blog. It turns out that on January 23 of last year Pants took her first steps since the surgery! I felt that the one-year anniversary of that momentous event deserved another just-as-momentous event (in fact, Jodi came downstairs shortly after me and had the same idea).

A LITTLE HISTORY...

During our last visit with Dr. Missiuna, he cleared her for all activities—except one. No trampoline! He also said her x-rays looked spectacular and that he wouldn't be seeing her for another twelve months. I thought one of us would have done a post back in December, but it seems we were too caught up in the holidays to boast about this wonderful news.

(Also, one thing I noticed about her x-rays was that there were no longer any gaps in her spine! Normally you would see vertebra—space—disc—space—vertebra—etc..., but in Pants's case it was just one big spine.)

Another thing was her upcoming class trip to the local ski hill. I signed up as a volunteer for this trip and had every intention of ensuring that I was never more than a few feet away from her the whole time. (Because what thirteen-year-old girl doesn't want her dad following her around on a class field trip?)

To say I was nervous about it was a bit of an understatement.

So, back to yesterday. Jodi and I decided that since the weather was nice and there was snow on the hill that I'd take Pants out for a couple hours of skiing and see how she made out. If she was shaky and needed a refresher

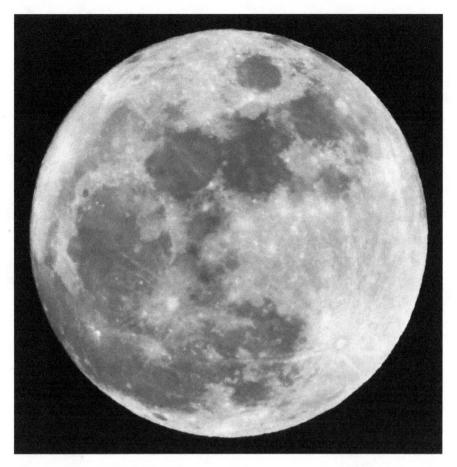

Avery's moon. (Andrew Butters)

lesson I'd sign her (us) up for one for one of the couple weekends prior to the ski outing with her class (and me).

Okay, so maybe it's one of those overprotective parent things, but at the top of the hill before our first run, I was ready to vomit. The good news is it only took Pants three turns before she felt right at home back on the slopes and well before the end of the day she was trying to find bumps to jump off. I even saw her catch a few inches of air once or twice. (More good news: I survived at least one or two heart attacks yesterday!)

She said to me afterwards, "I was nervous but after a few seconds my body was like, 'Hey, I remember how to do this!'"

ANDREW BUTTERS

After every run (which only took about a minute as the hills are small) she was positively beaming. Most of the time I could only see her eyes through her goggles and for three hours yesterday the only thing I saw was pure joy.

What a difference a year makes!

—Dad

P.S.

Last night as we were heading out to get burritos for dinner the most beautiful full moon was rising. After we ate dinner I ran out with my telescope and my Nikon and captured a few pics and declared that the first full moon of the New Year shall hereinafter be referred to as Avery's Moon.

168

FIFTEEN

THE REASON WE BLOGGED

Jodi started the blog because she found that there wasn't enough first-hand information about scoliosis on the internet. Sure, there were plenty of medical sites and lots of clinical papers. There were even a few woo-woo sites with fantastical claims about essential oils or other such "cures". But there wasn't much of anything that told the story from the patient's and from the family's perspective, certainly not a Canadian family.

Jodi, Avery and I were as open and candid as possible as we shared our thoughts, our fears, and our personal experiences with anyone who happened to stop by the blog and have a read. Then, one day almost one year since we started blogging I received an email message on Facebook.

September 11, 2015

Hi, I'm from Argentina and while searching for scoliosis surgery info, I found your blog. I immediately started to reading, post by post... I totally felt identified with your family's story. My fifteen-year-old son will take the surgery in December. We choose that month because is summer vacation here from school. But we heard all of this months ago. Gonzalo (that's my son's name) grew a lot these last months, and it was then we realised that his back was not straight. You can imagine how I feel about all this. Your blog helped me a lot, because I realized that other people have felt like myself.

Avery is a very brave girl, so sweet... congratulations to your family on my part and grateful that you have shared your experience with others who are going through the same situation.

Best wishes for your family :)

Carla

I would be lying if I said reading that email didn't bring a tear to my eye. I called Avery into the room right away and showed her. Her response was classic Avery.

AVERY: HELLO ARGENTINA!

September 13, 2015

Hello Argentina! I was heading up to bed, when my dad asked me to come and look at something. That something was a note/letter/post thingie from a person in Argentina about how they read our blog, and that their son was having the same surgery I had, but in December. After reading that, I got a bit sad that another person had to have the surgery, but I smiled really, really, big, because my family and I were helping people out, at least a bit, just by writing down our experiences. And now I am writing this post. Literally one minute ago I read the note thingie. I just wanted to say thank you.

I wish you luck, Gonzalo.

Until another day.

—Princess Pants

That kicked off a series of short posts in which Avery would send out her thoughts to Gonzalo. Avery and Gonzalo now follow each other on Instagram, as do I, and I am Facebook friends with both Gonzalo and his mother Carla.

Since that message from Carla came through I have given out the link to our blog easily a dozen times. Friends on Facebook or otherwise sent me a note asking if it was okay if they gave out my email address so they could pass it along to someone they know going through the same thing. Blog traffic has tapered since Avery, Jodi, and I stopped posting but it has also stayed consistent. People are still finding the site and they are still reading about our family's journey. You have managed to come this far and for that I thank you. There are, however, some questions that have yet to be answered. It is only fitting that I bring closure to those items and provide the best answers I can.

SIXTEEN

QUESTIONS ANSWERED

At the beginning of this journey I answered some questions such as: "What caused it?" and "How did you find out?" There were other questions that I didn't answer right away but instead answered through the blog posts from Avery, Jodi, and I. Here is a handy summary:

HOW LONG DID YOU HAVE TO WAIT FOR SURGERY?

From Avery's official diagnosis to Avery's surgery was 296 days. From first meeting with the surgeon to the actual surgery date was 256 days. From the time we were told Avery was next in line to the surgery date was 47 days. To give you some idea of how that compares to other kids in similar situations I can only give you wait times—times from when you are told you need surgery to the time the surgery takes place. In the province of Ontario here in Canada the wait times for this surgery vary and none of them are short. Toronto's Sick Kids has a wait time of 200 days. McMaster Children's Hospital where Avery's surgery took place has a wait time of 284 days. The Children's Hospital of Eastern Ontario (CHEO) has a wait time of 241 days. The provincial target set by the Ministry of Health is 182 days.

WAS AVERY SCARED?

Yes. Look back at a few of the posts from Avery. There is one she actually titled "I'm Scared" (January 3, 2015). That doesn't even begin to describe how terrified she was. Looking into her eyes as she lay on the table in the operating room there was nothing but fear. I talked with Avery as I put this book together and I asked her if she would look back and give me an idea of how scared she was. It's best if you read it for yourself:

"When I found out that my scoliosis had reached a stage where I needed surgery, I was terrified. For the first couple minutes I didn't quite understand, and it wasn't until we were leaving the hospital that it caught up with me. Before then I had been detached, and in an instant I was feeling too many emotions to understand any of them. There was fear, stemming from many worries. Anger that this was happening to me and sadness for the same reason, but mostly fear. Stomach-clenching, gut-wrenching fear. In between then and the day of the surgery there were good days and bad days, ups and downs, but everything was done with fear lurking in the back of my mind."

WERE YOU SCARED?

Yes, I was terrified.

For every one of the 256 days paralyzing fear was front and center. I had spoken with another parent whose daughter had a similar procedure but it didn't assuage my fears. I watched some videos of doctors explaining the surgery and it didn't help. I read entire websites devoted to this condition and I was still scared.

Maybe it is because I watch a lot of sports or maybe I heard the right analogy at the right time, but there was one moment where the fear I was carrying around wasn't all-consuming. Avery, Jodi, and I were seeing Dr. Missiuna for Avery's fourth appointment, which ended up being the last one before her pre-op visit to the hospital. Avery looked scared, I was scared, and Dr. Missiuna asked Avery a question. He asked, "How many times out of ten does a baseball player have to do his job correctly to be considered the best?" Avery didn't know much about baseball and said something like six or seven. Dr. Missiuna told her that it was somewhere between three and four. I could see the wheels turning inside Avery's head, and I had already made the connection, but hearing it for myself was the only thing throughout this experience that calmed my fears. I don't recall exactly what Dr. Missiuna said, but it was along the lines of, "Well my track record is perfect, and I intend to keep it that way."

That's all I needed to hear. I knew Dr. Missiuna was one of the best but I needed to hear him say it. This wasn't his first rodeo, as they say, and his track record to this point had nary a flaw. It was then that I realized that no matter how high my expectations of Dr. Missiuna were, his expectations of himself would always be higher.

I'm also certain that at least half of the calming talks that Dr. Missiuna had with Avery were as much for me as they were for Avery. I wear my emotions on my sleeve and hiding them has never been a strength of mine. That's why in the moment I was most afraid I hoped my acting skills were up to snuff.

When I was with Avery in the operating room I thought I was going to be sick. The only part of me that was visible were my eyes and I just hoped that Avery wouldn't recognize the paralyzing fear that had taken over my body. I asked her if she remembers anything from that moment and what she wrote brought a tear to my eye:

"On the operating table I often remember feeling safe. Now that I'm typing that it sounds like a weird thing to say, feeling safe before someone cuts you open, but it's true. There was fear in the background still, but I felt safe with my dad there, knowing that soon, in an instant for me, an eternity for my parents, and more than 24 hours for everyone else, I would be awake and fixed. I would be all better. So yes, I felt safe. I suppose it helped that I was being put under anaesthetic, as well."

WHAT EXACTLY DID THEY DO TO FIX IT?

Dr. Missiuna measured and cut two chrome/cobalt rods to the appropriate length—two inches (5.5cm) longer than her curved spine and then bent them into an optimal "model's posture." The rods are attached to her spine with 27 titanium screws. I don't know how long they are but by looking at the x-rays I'd say they were two inches. The screws sit in small holes that are drilled into each vertebra. The margin for error for each hole drilled is 1/64 of an inch (2mm). In Avery's case Dr. Missiuna did not drill one of the holes because he felt it was too risky. Then, a mixture of bone fragments and synthetic material was placed between her vertebrae and her disks (filling in the gaps). Over time this concoction hardens and new bone grows where the spaces used to be resulting in a rigid spine.

What remains when everything is all healed up is one solid spine with the metal hardware forever stuck in place. Extra support, if you will.

HOW LONG DOES IT TAKE TO HEAL?
WILL SHE BE ABLE TO DO EVERYTHING SHE DID BEFORE?

If you've read the book this far you can figure it out for yourself but I think a simple timeline will work best for answering this question:

Surgery
From the time I walked Avery into surgery to when she was wheeled up to the ICU was a little more than eleven hours.

In the Paediatric ICU
Avery spent less than one day in the ICU. For her, it was around twenty hours.

Post-Surgery Time in Hospital
From the time Avery left the ICU to the day her discharge papers were signed was six days.

Inactive at Home
Avery spent three weeks at home (four weeks post-surgery) before going to school for thirty minutes a day.

Back to School
It was a full seventeen weeks before Avery was back to school for the whole school day.

Light Activities
It was thirty-three weeks before Avery returned to yoga class.

Gym Class

It was nine months before Avery was cleared for activities like gym class but was not to participate in anything that made her feel uncomfortable. For example, burpees were struck from the list as they caused her pain.

All Clear!

It was eleven months before Avery was cleared for all activities except trampoline. Avery will never trampoline again. We are okay with this.

Will they ever take the rods out?

No. It is considered too risky to remove the hardware so, unless there is some malfunction or something is causing Avery a lot of pain the rods and screws will stay right where they are.

Finally, we have the most asked question (and I mean most by a landslide):

WILL SHE BEEP WHEN SHE GOES THROUGH AIRPORT SECURITY?

The answer we were given was "no". Chrome/cobalt and titanium are non-ferrous so conventional metal detectors won't pick them up. That being said, equipment is getting more and more sensitive, and new technology is developed every week, so who knows? We put this to the test thirteen months after Avery's surgery when the family took a much-deserved cruise around the Gulf of Mexico. Going through the metal detectors at Pearson International Airport before boarding our flight to Miami, Avery beeped.

In previous discussions with Dr. Missiuna Jodi and I asked if we should have a note from him indicating that Avery had metal rods attached to her spine. His response was quite on point. "If they need proof, just have Avery show them the scar!" So, when Avery beeped that's exactly what Jodi did, and off we went without any further issue.

Avery was on and off the ship several times, passing through a metal detector each time on the way back and didn't beep once, nor did she beep on the return flight from Miami to Orlando and Orlando back to Toronto. So, top marks go to Pearson International for their security screening!

SEVENTEEN

FINAL THOUGHTS

As you can see, Avery was fortunate enough to live where she lives and have access to the greatest, most affordable medical care one could hope for. Not a minute has passed since this incredible journey began that I haven't been thankful. There are too many people in this world who don't have access to, or can't afford, these miracles. Hopefully, from this book a friend will gain some insight, a parent will gain some confidence, or a child will gain some comfort just as Carla and Gonzalo from Argentina did.

Avery achieved the best possible outcome, but it was a heck of a journey. As I look back at everything I can share a few lessons that served Jodi and I quite well. Here are seven tips for parents to help get you ready and get you through surgery and walking side-by-side with your child on the road to recovery.

LEADING UP TO SURGERY
Give your child a voice
Before the surgery my daughter wouldn't talk much about her feelings. If she did she always seemed like she was trying to get an answer right on a test. I suppose that's the world she lives in, though. Answer a question, get a grade. Knowing the surgery was weighing on her, it was important she got the chance to express herself freely and without judgement. Whether it is through a blog, a journal, or a colouring book, I recommend you make sure your child has a

medium to communicate their feelings. Let them know they have a voice and give them the opportunity to use it.

Share your voice with your child

I sat down regularly with my daughter and asked her if she had written anything recently. I knew if she had or not, but it gave her the opportunity to try to articulate her feelings. Then, I shared my feelings with her. We discussed visualizations and meditation after yoga class and I told her all the things that worked for me. It was easy for me to think that sharing my fears would make things worse; that I needed to 'be strong' and 'show no fear,' but by not sharing my thoughts I was missing out on the perfect opportunity to show her ways to manage fear and it became something we acknowledged and dealt with together.

Count your blessings

Every time I found myself feeling depressed over the crappy hand we were dealt I also thought about how lucky my daughter was that she had a problem that could be fixed. It sounds terrible, but I had to constantly remind myself that there is always someone out there who is worse off. This wasn't an elective procedure. It was necessary for her health but in the end it would make her almost as good as new. Many children are not as fortunate and would gladly switch places. Also, my daughter was lucky that there was a team of incredibly skilled and dedicated healthcare professionals.

DURING SURGERY

Take care of yourself

The waiting was torture. I could barely stomach the simplest foods and I didn't want to drink too much and have to use the bathroom. What if I was needed for… something? What if something happened? I needed to be right there. My wife, who is much more pragmatic that I am encouraged me to use this time to rest, write emails to family or friends, blog, watch TV, or do whatever possible to try and remain calm. As hard as it was, eating was paramount. Strength and energy (mental and physical) are needed in epic proportions in times like these. Ensure your reserve tanks are filled to the brim.

Remember that no news is good news

If the surgery is scheduled for a long time it will be natural for you to wonder what is going on. I remember my wife constantly had to remind me that everyone in that operating room was doing their very best and if there was a concern that needed to be brought to our attention they would tell us. Remember all the incredible skill and dedication these healthcare professionals have? Yeah, they got this.

AFTER SURGERY

Put yourself in their shoes

The surgical team has done their part; now it's your child's time to do theirs. This is the perfect time to walk a mile in their shoes. Remember that they will be tired, confused, medicated, and likely in pain. Cut them some slack if they aren't the cheery, polite child you have worked so hard to raise. They've been through a lot and have healing to do. A little empathy goes a long way.

ALWAYS

Be there for them

When I asked Avery what was the best thing that Jodi and I did for her throughout her diagnosis, surgery, and recovery she said, "You were there for me."

You don't have to be perfect, but you do have to be present, and it will make all the difference in the world.

It means a lot to me that you took the time to follow this journey and I cannot thank you enough. If you or someone you know is following a similar path my thoughts and well-wishes are with you. Trust and thank your surgeon and health care support staff. Hug the ones you love.

—Dad

ACKNOWLEDGMENTS

I think if Avery, Jodi, and I thought about it we could write an entire novel just thanking everyone involved but I'll do my best to summarize. First of all, we have to thank Dr. Missiuna. His dedication to his field of expertise is shown through his dedication to his patients. He and his team pitched a perfect game when it came to straightening Avery out and have given her new life.

The support staff and extended health care team at McMaster Children's Hospital did an exemplary job with Avery as well as in supporting Jodi and I. World-class would be the best way to describe the dozens of doctors, nurses, physiotherapists, researchers, orderlies, and staff members at McMaster Children's. Thank you all for everything you did and continue to do day and night.

To our families, your love and support was immeasurable. You shared our fears and did your best to help relieve the burden. We are fortunate to have family members who are so loving.

Thank you to Stephanie for answering Avery's call when she had her fall, and for being an excellent caregiver to our little girl.

To our employers and coworkers and to all the teachers and students at Avery's school, your support through this made it possible for everyone to function and we thank you.

We can't say enough good things about Mike Chapman of Breathe Into

Motion Yoga Studios. Mike knows biomechanics, Mike knows yoga, and Mike has a heart ten sizes bigger than anyone we know. Namaste.

Andrew would like to thank all the wonderful people in his online writing group. They let him vent and cry and babble on, and were always there for him. They are the reason he was able to sit down and write about this experience without becoming an emotional puddle and this book would not be in print if it weren't for their collective wisdom.

Andrew also wants to thank his Brudder, Mama Bear, J-Gra, Mags, and his favourite wrestling tag-team champions of the world, Word Count and Writerghoulie. It is said that a person should surround themselves with greatness and each one of you fits that description to a "T".

Yes, Richard, Andrew should be writing.

We would also like to extend a thank you to Vance Joy, who didn't need to send Avery an autographed picture, but who did anyway, and included a handwritten note on top of that. You brought pure unadulterated joy to a girl who needed it.

To all of our friends on social media, you were a constant heartbeat of support. Thank you.

We would like to extend our gratitude to Carla and Gonzalo. Opening up and sharing your story with us changed the way we view the world. We are thrilled to know that you have made it through your journey as well as Avery made it through hers. You are proof positive that none of us is ever truly alone.

Finally, we would like to thank everyone who took the time to read a blog post or pick up this book. We hope that it has impacted you in a positive way. Reach out to us at any time if you have questions or want to share a story with us: bentbutnotbrokencanada@gmail.com

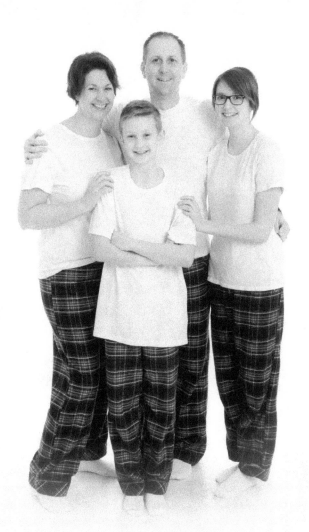

Andrew Butters has been in the software business since 1997, writing since 2010, and as the one who came up with the idea of turning the family blog chronicling their personal struggle with scoliosis into a book to help other families through their own.

Avery Butters was born in 2002 and diagnosed with scoliosis in 2014 at the age of 12 after a routine exam. This is her story. Her younger brother, AJ Butters, was born in 2006, and was the reason Avery's condition was uncovered.

Jodi Wilks-Butters has been a public servant since 1996, and the original blog that gave rise to Bent But Not Broken was her idea.

They all live together in southwestern Ontario, Canada with their three cats.

www.bentbutnotbroken.net